FV

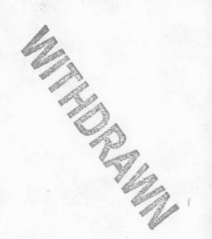

WITHDRAWN

SKIN SHOWS

SKIN

Gothic Horror and the Technology of Monsters

SHOWS

Judith Halberstam

Duke University Press   Durham and London 1995

© 1995 Duke University Press
All rights reserved
Printed in the United States of America on acid-free paper ∞
Typeset in Galliard by Keystone Typesetting, Inc.
Library of Congress Cataloging-in-Publication Data appear
on the last printed page of this book.

This book is dedicated to
Heini and Doreen Halberstam

Contents

Acknowledgments

My thanks to many people who have helped with this monster. In its earliest stages I benefited from the wisdom and advice of Nancy Armstrong and Leonard Tennenhouse, Jane Gallop, Paula Rabinowitz, Marty Roth, John Mowitt, and Susan McClary. As its size and proportions changed and grew, I was assisted intellectually and in other ways by many of my colleagues at the University of California at San Diego, especially Michael Davidson, Page DuBois, Lisa Lowe, Rosemary George, Kathryn Shevelow, and Winnie Woodhull. My editor, Ken Wissoker, and readers George Haggerty and particularly Ann Cvetkovich helped me to shape this into a much better book. Numerous students have contributed to this project but I want to especially thank my Graduate Seminar on Gender and the Horror Film for working through ideas with me. The University of Minnesota at Minneapolis supported this work with a travel grant and a dissertation fellowship. The University of California at San Diego generously assisted this project with Academic Senate travel grants and faculty fellowships. My co-conspirator in monster-making, Ira Livingston, shared bullets, buffaloes, junkyards and fast times in Missoula, Montana, with me. Thanks to friends for support and suggestions: Laura Harris, Jenni Olson, Elspeth Probyn, Sandy Stone, Heather Findlay, David Lloyd, Chandan Reddy, Katrin Seig, Michael Yamamoto. Special thanks to D. B. for dancing and other inappropriate delights. And finally, I want to express my gratitude to Barbara Cruikshank who graciously and lovingly put up with my own particular monstrosities through most of the writing of this book.

Chapter 4, "Technologies of Monstrosity: Bram Stoker's *Dracula*," originally appeared in *Victorian Studies* 36, no. 3 (Spring 1993): 333–352; an earlier version of chapter 7, "Skinflick: Posthuman Gender in Jonathan Demme's *The Silence of the Lambs*," appeared in *Camera Obscura* 27 (September 1991): 37–54.

SKIN SHOWS

Parasites and Perverts: An Introduction to Gothic Monstrosity

So many monsters; so little time.
—promotional slogan for HELLRAISER

Skin Shows

In *The Silence of the Lambs* (1991) by Jonathan Demme, one of many modern adaptations of *Frankenstein,* a serial killer known as Buffalo Bill collects women in order to flay them and use their skins to construct a "woman suit." Sitting in his basement sewing hides, Buffalo Bill makes his monster a sutured beast, a patchwork of gender, sex, and sexuality. Skin, in this morbid scene, represents the monstrosity of surfaces and as Buffalo Bill dresses up in his suit and prances in front of the mirror, he becomes a layered body, a body of many surfaces laid one upon the other. Depth and essence dissolve in this mirror dance and identity and humanity become skin deep.

My subject is monsters and I begin in Buffalo Bill's basement, his "filthy workshop of creation," because it dramatizes precisely the distance traveled between current representations of monstrosity and their genesis in nineteenth-century Gothic fiction. Where the monsters of the nineteenth century metaphorized modern subjectivity as a balancing act between inside/outside, female/male, body/mind, native/foreign, proletarian/aristocrat, monstrosity in postmodern horror films finds its place in what Baudrillard has called the obscenity of "immediate visibility"[1] and what Linda Williams has dubbed "the frenzy of the visible."[2] The immediate visibility of a Buffalo Bill, the way in which he makes the surface itself monstrous transforms the cavernous monstrosity of Jekyll/ Hyde, Dorian Gray, or Dracula into a beast who is all body and no soul.

Victorian monsters produced and were produced by an emergent conception of the self as a body which enveloped a soul, as a body, indeed, enthralled to its soul. Michel Foucault writes in *Discipline and Punish* that "the soul is the prison of the body" and he proposes a genealogy of the soul that will show it to be born out of "methods of punishment, supervision and constraint."[3] Foucault also claims that, as modern forms of discipline shifted their gaze from the body to the soul, crime literature moved from confession or gallows speeches or the cataloguing of famous criminals to the detective fiction obsessed with identifying criminality and investigating crime. The hero of such literature was now the middle- or upper-class schemer whose crime became a virtuoso performance of skill and enterprise.

There are many congruities between Gothic fiction and detective fiction but in the Gothic, crime is embodied within a specifically deviant form — the monster — that announces itself (de-monstrates) as the place of corruption. Furthermore, just as the detective character appears across genres in many different kinds of fiction (in the sensation novel, in Dickens), so Gothic infiltrates the Victorian novel as a symptomatic moment in which boundaries between good and evil, health and perversity, crime and punishment, truth and deception, inside and outside dissolve and threaten the integrity of the narrative itself. While many literary histories, therefore, have relegated Gothic to a subordinate status in relation to realism, I will be arguing that nineteenth-century literary tradition *is* a Gothic tradition and that this has everything to do with the changing technologies of subjectivity that Foucault describes.

Gothic fiction is a technology of subjectivity, one which produces the deviant subjectivities opposite which the normal, the healthy, and the pure can be known. Gothic, within my analysis, may be loosely defined as the rhetorical style and narrative structure designed to produce fear and desire within the reader. The production of fear in a literary text (as opposed to a cinematic text) emanates from a vertiginous excess of meaning. Gothic, in a way, refers to an ornamental excess (think of Gothic architecture — gargoyles and crazy loops and spirals), a rhetorical extravagance that produces, quite simply, too much. Within Gothic novels, I argue, multiple interpretations are embedded in the text and part of the experience of horror comes from the realization that meaning itself runs riot. Gothic novels produce a symbol for this interpretive mayhem in the body of the monster. The monster always becomes a primary focus of interpretation and its monstrosity seems available for any number of meanings. While I will examine closely the implications of embodied horror (monstrosity) in nineteenth-century Gothic, I will also be paying careful attention to the rhetorical system which produces it (Gothic).

Many histories of the Gothic novel begin with the Gothic Romances of the later eighteenth century by Mrs. Radcliffe, Horace Walpole, and Matthew Lewis.[4] While, obviously, there are connections to be made between these stories of mad monks, haunted castles, and wicked foreigners and the nineteenth-century Gothic tales of monsters and vampires, we should not take the connections too far. I will argue in this book that the emergence of the monster within Gothic fiction marks a peculiarly modern emphasis upon the horror of particular kinds of bodies. Furthermore, the ability of the Gothic story to take the imprint of any number of interpretations makes it a hideous offspring of capitalism itself. The Gothic novel of the nineteenth century and the Gothic horror film of the late twentieth century are both obsessed with multiple modes of consumption and production, with dangerous consumptions and excessive productivity, and with economies of meaning. The monster itself is an economic form in that it condenses various racial and sexual threats to nation, capitalism, and the bourgeoisie in one body. If the Gothic novel produces an easy answer to the question of what threatens national security and prosperity (the monster), the Gothic monster represents many answers to the question of who must be removed from the community at large. I will be considering, therefore, nineteenth- and twentieth-century Gothic as separate from eighteenth-century Gothic, but I will also be tracing Gothic textuality across many modes of discourse.

Within the nineteenth-century Gothic, authors mixed and matched a wide variety of signifiers of difference to fabricate the deviant body — Dracula, Jekyll/Hyde, and even Frankenstein's monster before them are lumpen bodies, bodies pieced together out of the fabric of race, class, gender, and sexuality. In the modern period and with the advent of cinematic body horror, the shift from the literary Gothic to the visual Gothic was accompanied by a narrowing rather than a broadening of the scope of horror. One might expect to find that cinema multiplies the possibilities for monstrosity but in fact, the visual register quickly reaches a limit of visibility. In *Frankenstein* the reader can only imagine the dreadful spectacle of the monster and so its monstrosity is limited only by the reader's imagination; in the horror film, the monster must always fail to be monstrous enough and horror therefore depends upon the explicit violation of female bodies as opposed to simply the sight of the monster.

Furthermore, as I noted, while nineteenth-century Gothic monstrosity was a combination of the features of deviant race, class, and gender, within contemporary horror, the monster, for various reasons, tends to show clearly the markings of deviant sexualities and gendering but less clearly the signs of class or race. Buffalo Bill in *The Silence of the Lambs,* for example, leads one to suppose that the monstrous body is a sexed or gendered body only, but this particular body, a borrowed skin, is also clearly inscribed with a narrative of class conflict. To give just one example of deviant class in this film, the heroine, Clarice Starling, is identified by Hannibal Lecter as a woman trying to hide her working-class roots behind "bad perfume" and cheap leather shoes. Given the emphases in this film upon skins and hides, it is all too significant that cheap leather gives Starling away. Poor skin, in this film, literally signifies poverty, or the trace of it. As we will see, however, the narrative of monstrous class identity has been almost completely subsumed within *The Silence of the Lambs* by monstrous sexuality and gender.

The discourse of racialized monstrosity within the modern horror film proves to be a discursive minefield. Perhaps because race has been so successfully gothicized within our recent history, filmmakers and screenplay writers tend not to want to make a monster who is defined by a deviant racial identity. European anti-Semitism and American racism towards black Americans are precisely Gothic discourses given over to the making monstrous of particular kinds of bodies. This study will de-lineate carefully the multiple strands of anti-Semitism within nineteenth-century Gothic and I will attempt to suggest why anti-Semitism in par-ticular used Gothic methods to make Jews monstrous. But when it comes to tracing the threads of Gothic race into modern horror, we often draw a blank.

The gothicization of certain "races" over the last century, one might say, has been all too successful. This does not mean that Gothic race is not readable in the contemporary horror text but it is clear that, within Gothic, the difference between representing racism and representing race is extremely tricky to negotiate. I will be arguing, in relation to *The Silence of the Lambs,* that the film clearly represents homophobia and sexism and punishes actions motivated by them; it would be very diffi-cult in a horror film to show and punish racism simultaneously. To give an example of what I am arguing here, one can look at a contemporary horror film, *Candyman* (1990), and the way it merges monstrosity and race.

In *Candyman* two female graduate students in anthropology at the

University of Illinois at Chicago are researching urban legends when they run across the story of Candyman, the ghost of a murdered black man who haunts the Cabrini Green projects. Candyman was the son of a former slave who made good by inventing a procedure for the mass production of shoes. Despite his wealth, Candyman still ran into trouble with the white community by falling in love with a white woman. He was chased by white men to Cabrini Green where they caught him, cut his right hand off, and drove a hook into the bloody stump. Next Candyman was covered in honey and taken to an apiary where the bees killed him. Now, the urban myth goes, Candyman responds to all who call him. The two researchers, a white woman and a black woman, go to Cabrini Green to hunt for information on Candyman. Naturally, the black woman, Bernadette, is killed by Candyman, and the white woman, Helen, is seduced by him. While the film on some level attempts to direct all kinds of social criticisms at urban planners, historians, and racist white homeowners, ultimately the horror stabilizes in the ghastly body of the black man whose monstrosity turns upon his desire for the white woman and his murderous intentions towards black women.

No amount of elaborate framing within this film can prevent it from confirming racist assumptions about black male aggression towards white female bodies. Monstrosity, in this tired narrative, never becomes mobile; rather, it remains anchored by the weight of racist narratives. The film contains some clever visual moves, like a shot of Helen going through the back of a mirror into a derelict apartment. She next passes through a hole in the wall and the camera reverses to show her stepping through a graffiti painting of a black man's face. She stops for a moment in the mouth of the black man and this startling image hints at the various forms of oral transmissions that the film circulates. Is Helen contained by the oral history of the Candyman or is she the articulate voice of the academy that disrupts its transmission and brings violence to the surface? Inevitably, Helen's character stabilizes under the sign of the white woman victim and Candyman's horror becomes a static signifier of black male violence. If race in nineteenth-century Gothic was one of many clashing surfaces of monstrosity, in the context of twentieth-century Gothic, race becomes a master signifier of monstrosity and when invoked, it blocks out all other possibilities of monstrous identity.

Moving from nineteenth-century Gothic monsters to the monsters of contemporary horror films, my study will show that within the history of embodied deviance, monsters always combine the markings of a plurality of differences even if certain forms of difference are eclipsed momentarily by others. The fact that monstrosity within contemporary horror seems to have stabilized into an amalgam of sex and gender demonstrates the need to read a history of otherness into and out of the history of Gothic fiction. Gothic fiction of the nineteenth century specifically used the body of the monster to produce race, class, gender, and sexuality within narratives about the relation between subjectivities and certain bodies.

Monstrosity (and the fear it gives rise to) is historically conditioned rather than a psychological universal. Tracing the emergence of monstrosity from *Frankenstein* through to the contemporary horror film (in both its high- and low-budget forms), I will attempt to show that monsters not only reveal certain material conditions of the production of horror, but they also make strange the categories of beauty, humanity, and identity that we still cling to. While the horror within *Frankenstein* seemed to depend upon the monster's actual hideous physical aspect, his status as anomaly, and his essential foreignness, the threat of Buffalo Bill depends upon the violence of his identity crisis, a crisis that will exact a price in female flesh. Buffalo Bill's identity crisis is precisely that, a crisis of knowledge, a "category crisis"[5]; but it no longer takes the form of the anomaly—now a category crisis indicates a crisis of sexual identity.

It is in the realm of sexuality, however, that Buffalo Bill and Frankenstein's monster seem to share traits and it is here that we may be inclined to read Buffalo Bill as a reincarnation of many of the features of nineteenth-century monstrosity. As a sexual being, Frankenstein's monster is foreign and as an outsider to the community, his foreign sexuality is monstrous and threatens miscegenation. Frankenstein's lonely monster is driven out of town by the mob when he threatens to reproduce. Similarly, Buffalo Bill threatens the community with his indeterminate gender and sexuality. Indeed, sexuality and its uneasy relation to gender identity creates Buffalo Bill's monstrosity. But much ground has been traveled between the stitched monstrosity of Frankenstein and the sutured gender horror of Buffalo Bill; while both monsters have been sewn into skin bodysuits and while both want to jump out of their skins, the nineteenth-century monster is marked by racial or species violation while Buffalo Bill seems to be all gender. If we measure one skin job against the other, we can read transitions between various signifying systems of identity.

Skin, I will argue with reference to certain nineteenth-century monsters, becomes a kind of metonym for the human; and its color, its pallor, its shape mean everything within a semiotic of monstrosity. Skin might be too tight (Frankenstein's creature), too dark (Hyde), too pale (Dracula), too superficial (Dorian Gray's canvas), too loose (Leatherface), or too sexed (Buffalo Bill). Skin houses the body and it is figured in Gothic as the ultimate boundary, the material that divides the inside from the outside. The vampire will puncture and mark the skin with his fangs, Mr. Hyde will covet white skin, Dorian Gray will desire his own canvas, Buffalo Bill will covet female skin, Leatherface will wear his victim's skin as a trophy and recycle his flesh as food. Slowly but surely the outside becomes the inside and the hide no longer conceals or contains, it offers itself up as text, as body, as monster. The Gothic text, whether novel or film, plays out an elaborate skin show.

How sexuality became the dominant mark of otherness is a question that we may begin to answer by deconstructing Victorian Gothic monsters and examining the constitutive features of the horror they represent. If, for example, many nineteenth-century monsters seem to produce fears more clearly related to racial identity than gender identity, how is it that we as modern readers have been unable to discern these more intricate contours of difference? Obviously, the answer to such a question and many others like it lies in a history of sexuality, a history introduced by Michel Foucault and continued by recent studies which link Foucault's work to a history of the novel.[6]

In this study I am not simply attempting to add racial, national, or class difference to the already well-defined otherness of sexual perversion nor am I attempting merely another reading of the Gothic tradition; I am suggesting that, where the foreign and the sexual merge within monstrosity in Gothic, a particular history of sexuality unfolds. It is indeed necessary to map out a relation between the monstrous sexuality of the foreigner and the foreign sexuality of the monster because sexuality, I will argue, is itself a beast created in nineteenth-century literature. Where sexuality becomes an identity, other "others" become invisible and the multiple features of monstrosity seem to degenerate back into a primeval sexual slime. Class, race, and nation are subsumed, in other words, within the monstrous sexual body; accordingly, Dracula's bite drains pleasure rather than capital, Mr. Hyde symbolizes repression rather than the production of self, and both figure foreign aspect as a threat to domestic security. While I will attempt here to delineate the mechanism by which multiple otherness is subsumed by the unitary otherness of sexuality, it is actually beyond the scope of this study to account for the very particular and individual histories of race, nation, and class within the nineteenth century. I am concerned specifically with representational strategies and with the particularities of deviant race, class, national and gender markings.

Past studies of the Gothic have tended toward the psychological, or more precisely, the psychoanalytic, because the unconscious is assumed to be the proper seat of fear. So, for example, there are studies of the Gothic which associate Gothic with masochism,[7] with the abject maternal,[8] with women's "fear of self,"[9] with the very construction of female identity.[10] And yet, as critics like Michel Foucault and Gilles Deleuze and Félix Guattari have shown, the unconscious itself and all of its mechanisms are precisely the effects of historical and cultural production. Therefore, to historicize monstrosity in literature, and especially in the Gothic novel, reveals a specificity within the way that, since the age of Frankenstein and Dracula, monsters mark difference within and upon bodies. A historical study of Gothic and of Gothic monstrosity must actually avoid psychoanalytic readings just long enough to expose the way that Gothic actually participates in the production of something like a psychology of self. However, as will be clear, certain psychoanalytic positions on fear and desire are useful ways of negotiating between the psychic and the social and of showing how some social mechanisms are internalized to the point that they are experienced as internal mechanisms. In order to examine such a process, a detour through Freud's case histories of paranoia will be necessary.

The body that scares and appalls changes over time, as do the individual characteristics that add up to monstrosity, as do the preferred interpretations of that monstrosity. Within the traits that make a body monstrous — that is, frightening or ugly, abnormal or disgusting — we may read the difference between an other and a self, a pervert and a normal person, a foreigner and a native. Furthermore, in order to read monsters as the embodiments of psychic horror, one must first of all subscribe to psychoanalysis's own tale of human subjectivity — a fiction intent upon rewriting the Gothic elements of human subjectivity. As I have said, my study refuses the universality of what Deleuze and Guattari call the "daddy-mommy-me triangle"[11] but it cannot always escape the triangle. With characteristic grim humor, Deleuze and Guattari describe the psychoanalytic encounter between analyst and patient: "The psycho-analyst no longer says to the patient: 'Tell me a little bit about your desiring machines, won't you?' Instead he screams: 'Answer daddy-and-mommy when I speak to you!' Even Melanie Klein. So the entire process of desiring-production is trampled underfoot and reduced to parental images, laid out step by step in accordance with supposed pre-oedipal stages, totalized in Oedipus. . . ."[12] Within modern Western culture, we are disciplined through a variety of social and political mechanisms into psychoanalytic relations and then psychoanalytic explanations are deployed to totalize our submission. Resistance in such a circular system, as many theorists have noted, merely becomes part of the oppressive mechanism. However, as we will see in later chapters of this study, psychoanalysis, with its emphases on and investments in the normal, quickly reveals itself to be inadequate to the task of unraveling the power of horror.

In relation to Gothic monstrosity, it is all too easy to understand how the relation between fear and desire may be oedipalized, psychologized, humanized. Psychoanalysis itself has a clinical term for the transformation of desire into fear and of the desired/feared object into monster: paranoia. Freud believed that his theory of paranoia as a repressed homosexual desire could be applied to any and all cases of paranoia regardless of race or social class. This, of course, is where the psychoanalytic crisis begins and ends — in its attempt to reduce everything to the sexual and then in its equation of sexuality and identity. The process by which political material becomes sexual material is one in which the novel plays a major role. And the Gothic novel, particularly the late-Victorian Gothic novel, provides a metaphor for this process in the form of the monster. The monster is the product of and the symbol for the transformation of identity into sexual identity through the mechanism of failed repression.

One Lacanian account of monstrosity demonstrates simultaneously the appeal and the danger of psychoanalytic explanations. In Slavoj Žižek's essay "Grimaces of the Real, Or When the Phallus Appears," he reads the phantom from *The Phantom of the Opera* alongside such enigmatic images as the vampire, Edvard Munch's *The Scream* (1893), and David Lynch's *Elephant Man* (1980).[13] Žižek attempts to position images of the living-dead as both mediators between high art and mass culture and as "the void of the pure self" (67). Žižek is at his most persuasive when he discusses the multiplicity of meaning generated by the monster. The fecundity of the monster as a symbol leads him to state: "The crucial question is not 'What does the phantom signify?' but

'How is the very space constituted where entities like the phantom can emerge?'" (63). The monster/phantom, in other words, never stands for a simple or unitary prejudice, it always acts as a "fantasy screen" upon which viewers and readers inscribe and sexualize meaning.

Žižek also seems to be very aware of the dangers of what he calls "the so-called psychoanalytic interpretation of art" which operates within a kind of spiral of interpretation so that everything *means* psychoanalysis. Accordingly, rather than explain the mother's voice in *Psycho* as the maternal superego, he suggests "turn(ing) it around, to explain the very logic of the maternal superego by means of this vocal stain" (51). But Žižek does not always sustain his challenge to the hegemonic structure of psychoanalysis. Indeed, he often stays firmly within the interpretive confines of the psychoanalytic model and merely uses cultural texts as examples of psychoanalytic functions (particularly Lacanian functions). Within this model, the phantom of the opera, for example, is a "fetish," it literally stands in for various kinds of antagonisms: class-based, racial, economic, national, etc. But the fetish remains always a sexual mechanism and this is where Žižek's analysis is doomed to reproduce the process which it attempts to explain; the fetish is a sexualized object that stands in for and indeed covers up other kinds of antagonism. Žižek gives, as an example of the fetishistic role of the phantom, the Jew of anti-Semitic discourse. While this book will also make concrete connections between anti-Semitism and the Gothic production of monsters and indeed, between racial and sexual layers of signification, it is crucial to an interpretation of Gothic to understand that the Jew/phantom/monster is sexualized within fictional narratives (and this includes pseudo-scientific and social-scientific narratives that are usually classified as nonfiction) as a part of the narrative process that transforms class/race/gender threat into sexual threat.

Žižek's claim, then, that "the Jew is the anal object par excellence, that is to say, the partial object stain that disturbs the harmony of the class relationship" (57) precisely leaves intact the sexualization of Jewishness; his assertion that the phantom of the living-dead is the emergence of "the anal father" or "primal father" and the opposite of paternal law reinscribes parental (symbolic or otherwise) relations into a scene that precisely seems to escape the familial; his claim, finally, that vampires do not appear in mirrors because "they have read their Lacan" and know, therefore, that "they materialize object *a* which, by definition, *cannot be mirrored*" (55), begs to be read as a parody of what it invokes but instead actually continues to posit subjects that simply do not exist independent of their production in Lacanian psychoanalysis.

The vampire of the nineteenth-century narrative has most certainly not read his/her Lacan (*avant la lettre*) and does not know that he/she cannot be mirrored. This vampire crawls face down along the wall dividing self from other, class from race from gender and drains metaphoricity from one place only to infuse it in another. While Žižek claims often in his work to be using psychoanalysis and specifically Lacan to explain popular culture paradigms, too often he merely uses popular culture to explain Lacan. And, of course, this particular relationship between host and parasite is the only one that psychoanalytic discourse can endorse. Žižek warns: "The analysis that focuses on the 'ideological meaning' of monsters overlooks the fact that, before signifying something, before serving as a vessel of meaning, monsters embody enjoyment qua the limit of interpretation, that is to say, *nonmeaning as such*" (64). The idea that a realm of "nonmeaning" exists prior to interpretation is only possible in a structural universe in which form and content can easily be separated. Gothic literature in particular is a rhetorical form which resists the disintegration of form and content.[14] Monstrosity always unites monstrous form with monstrous meaning.

In *Skin Shows* I will be situating Gothic as a site or topos in nineteenth-century fiction and contemporary horror film. In its typical form, the Gothic topos is the monstrous body à la Frankenstein, Dracula, Dorian Gray, Jekyll/Hyde; in its generic form, Gothic is the disruption of realism and of all generic purity. It is the hideous eruption of the monstrous in the heart of domestic England but it is also the narrative that calls genre itself into question. Mary Shelley's *Frankenstein,* which I think functions as an allegory of Gothic production, contains a domestic tableau of family life (the De Laceys) right in the heart of the narrative. This structure inverts and threatens to maintain a reversal whereby, rather than the Gothic residing in the dark corners of realism, the realistic is buried alive in the gloomy recesses of Gothic. It may well be that the novel is always Gothic.

Gothic Gnomes

In her 1832 introduction to *Frankenstein,* Shelley writes, "I bid my hideous progeny go forth and prosper."[15] Shelley's "hideous progeny" was not merely her novel but the nineteenth-century Gothic novel itself.

The Gothic, of course, did indeed prosper and thrive through the century. It grew in popularity until, by the turn of the century, its readership was massive enough that a writer could actually make a living from the sale of his Gothic works. In 1891, for example, Robert Louis Stevenson loosed his "shilling shocker," *Dr. Jekyll and Mr. Hyde,* upon the reading public hoping for commercial returns. Stevenson described his novella as a "Gothic gnome" and worried that he had produced a gross distortion of literature.[16] Such an anxiety marked Gothic itself as a monstrous form in relation to its popularity and its improper subject matter. The appellation "Gothic gnome" labeled the genre as a mutation or hybrid form of true art and genteel literature.

But monsters do indeed sell books and books sell monsters and the very popularity of the Gothic suggests that readers and writers collaborate in the production of the features of monstrosity. Gothic novels, in fact, thematize the monstrous aspects of both production and consumption — *Frankenstein* is, after all, an allegory about a production that refuses to submit to its author and *Dracula* is a novel about an archconsumer, the vampire, who feeds upon middle-class women and then turns them into vampires by forcing them to feed upon him. The Gothic, in fact, like the vampire itself, creates a public who consumes monstrosity, who revels in it, and who then surveys its individual members for signs of deviance or monstrosity, excess or violence.

Anxiety about the effects of consuming popular literature revealed itself in England in the 1890s in the form of essays and books which denounced certain works as "degenerate" (a label defined by Max Nordau's book *Degeneration*).[17] Although Gothic fiction obviously fell into this category, the censors missed the mark in denouncing such works. Rather than condoning the perversity they recorded, Gothic authors, in fact, seemed quite scrupulous about taking a moral stand against the unnatural acts that produce monstrosity. Long sentimental sermons on truth and purity punctuate many a gruesome tale and leave few doubts as to its morality by the narrative's end. Bram Stoker, for example, sermonizes both in his novels and in an essay printed in the journal *The Nineteenth Century* called "The Censorship of Fiction." In this essay, Stoker calls for stricter surveillance of popular fiction and drama. Stoker thinks censorship would combat human weakness on two levels, namely, "the weakness of the great mass of people who form audiences, and of those who are content to do base things in the way of catering for these base appetites."[18] Obviously, Stoker did not expect his own writing to be received as a work that "catered to base appetites" because, presumably, it used perverse sexuality to identify what or who threatened the dominant class.

Similarly, Oscar Wilde was shocked by the critics who called *The Picture of Dorian Gray* "poisonous" and "heavy with the mephitic odours of moral and spiritual putrefaction." Wilde's novel, after all, tells the story of a young man seduced by a poisonous book and punished soundly for his corruptions. Wilde defends his work by saying, "It was necessary, sir, for the dramatic development of this story to surround Dorian Gray with an atmosphere of moral corruption." He continues, "Each man sees his own sin in Dorian Gray."[19]

Producing and consuming monsters and monstrous fictions, we might say, adds up to what Eve Sedgwick has called, in her study of Gothic conventions, "an aesthetic of pleasurable fear."[20] The Gothic, in other words, inspires fear and desire at the same time — fear of and desire for the other, fear of and desire for the possibly latent perversity lurking within the reader herself. But fear and desire within the same body produce a disciplinary effect. In other words, a Victorian public could consume Gothic novels in vast quantities without regarding such a material as debased because Gothic gave readers the thrill of reading about so-called perverse activities while identifying aberrant sexuality as a condition of otherness and as an essential trait of foreign bodies. The monster, of course, marks the distance between the perverse and the supposedly disciplined sexuality of a reader. Also, the signifiers of "normal" sexuality maintain a kind of hegemonic power by remaining invisible.

So, the aesthetic of pleasurable fear that Sedgwick refers to makes pleasure possible only by fixing horror elsewhere, in an obviously and literally foreign body, and by then articulating the need to expel the foreign body. Thus, both Dracula and Hyde are characters with markedly foreign physiognomies; they are dark and venal, foreign in both aspect and behavior. Dracula, for example, is described by Harker as an angular figure with a strong face notable for "peculiarly arched nostrils . . . a lofty domed forehead," bushy hair and eyebrows, "sharp white teeth," and ears pointed at the tops.[21] Hyde is described as small and deformed, "pale and dwarfish . . . troglodytic."[22] By making monstrosity so obviously a physical condition and by linking it to sexual corruption, such fictions bind foreign aspects to perverse activities.

The most telling example I can find of a monstrous foreigner in Gothic is Bram Stoker's Count Dracula who obviously comes to England from a distant "elsewhere" in search of English blood. Critics have discussed at length the perverse and dangerous sexuality exhibited by the vampire but, with a few exceptions, criticism has not connected Dracula's sexual attacks with the threat of the foreign. Dracula, I argue in my fourth chapter, condenses the xenophobia of Gothic fiction into a very specific horror — the vampire embodies and exhibits all the stereotyping of nineteenth-century anti-Semitism. The anatomy of the vampire, for example, compares remarkably to anti-Semitic studies of Jewish physiognomy — peculiar nose, pointed ears, sharp teeth, claw-like hands — and furthermore, in Stoker's novel, blood and money (central facets in anti-Semitism) mark the corruption of the vampire. The vampire merges Jewishness and monstrosity and represents this hybrid monster as a threat to Englishness and English womanhood in particular. In the Jew, then, Gothic fiction finds a monster versatile enough to represent fears about race, nation, and sexuality, a monster who combines in one body fears of the foreign and the perverse.

Perversion and Parasitism

Within nineteenth-century anti-Semitism, the Jew was marked as a threat to capital, to masculinity, and to nationhood. Jews in England at the turn of the century were the objects of an internal colonization. While the black African became the threatening other abroad, it was closer to home that people focused their real fears about the collapse of nation through a desire for racial homogeneity.[23] Jews were referred to as "degenerate," the bearers of syphilis, hysterical, neurotic, as bloodsuckers and, on a more practical level, Jews were viewed as middlemen in business.[24] Not all Gothic novels are as explicit as *Dracula* about their identification of monster and Jew. In some works we can read a more generalized code of fear which links horror to the Oriental[25] and in others we must interpret a bodily semiotic that marks monsters as symbols of a diseased culture. But to understand better how the history of the Gothic novel charts the entanglement of race, nation, and sexuality in productions of otherness, we might consider the Gothic monster as the antithesis of "Englishness."

Benedict Anderson has written about the cultural roots of the nation in terms of "imagined communities" which are "conceived in language, not in blood."[26] By linking the development of a print industry, particularly the popularization of novels and newspapers, to the spread of nationalism, Anderson pays close attention to the ways in which a shared conception of what constitutes "nation-ness" is written and read across certain communities. If the nation, therefore, is a textual production which creates national community in terms of an inside and an outside and then makes those categories indispensable, Gothic becomes one place to look for a fiction of the foreign, a narrative of who and what is not-English and not-native. The racism that becomes a mark of nineteenth-century Gothic arises out of the attempt within horror fiction to give form to what terrifies the national community. Gothic monsters are defined both as other than the imagined community and as the being that cannot be imagined as community.

"Racism and anti-Semitism," Anderson writes, "manifest themselves, not across national boundaries, but within them. In other words, they justify not so much foreign wars as domestic oppression and domination" (136). The racism and anti-Semitism that I have identified as a hallmark of nineteenth-century Gothic literature certainly direct themselves towards a domestic rather than a foreign scene. Gothic in the 1890s, as represented by the works of Robert Louis Stevenson, Bram Stoker, and Oscar Wilde, takes place in the backstreets of London in laboratories and asylums, in old abandoned houses and decaying city streets, in hospitals and bedrooms, in homes and gardens. The monster, such a narrative suggests, will find you in the intimacy of your own home; indeed, it will make your home its home (or you its home) and alter forever the comfort of domestic privacy. The monster peeps through the window, enters through the back door, and sits beside you in the parlor; the monster is always invited in but never asked to stay. The racism that seems to inhere to the nineteenth-century Gothic monster, then, may be drawn from imperialistic or colonialist fantasies of other lands and peoples, but it concentrates its imaginative force upon the other peoples in "our" lands, the monsters at home. The figure of the parasite becomes paramount within Gothic precisely because it is an internal not an external danger that Gothic identifies and attempts to dispel.

In *The Origins of Totalitarianism*, Hannah Arendt has argued convincingly that the modern category of anti-Semitism emerges from both nineteenth-century attempts to make race the "key to history" and the particular history of the Jews as "a people without a government, without a country, and without a language."[27] As such, the Jew, with regards to nation and, for our purposes, to English nationality, might be said to represent the not-English, the not-middle-class, the parasitical tribe that drains but never restores or produces. Arendt shows how the decline of the aristocracy and of nationalism by the mid-nineteenth century made people seek new ground for both commonality and superiority. She writes, "For if race doctrines finally served more sinister and immediately political purposes, it is still true that much of their plausibility and persuasiveness lay in the fact that they helped anybody feel himself an aristocrat who had been selected by birth on the strength of 'racial' qualification." Arendt's point is of central importance to an understanding of the history of Gothic. We might note in passing that, from the late eighteenth century to the nineteenth century, the terrain of Gothic horror shifted from the fear of corrupted aristocracy or clergy, represented by the haunted castle or abbey, to the fear embodied by monstrous bodies. Reading Gothic with nineteenth-century ideologies of race suggests why this shift occurs. If, then, with the rise of bourgeois culture, aristocratic heritage became less and less of an index of essential national identity, the construction of national unity increasingly depended upon the category of race and class. Therefore, the blood of nobility now became the blood of the native and both were identified in contradistinction to so-called "impure" races such as Jews and Gypsies. The nobility, furthermore, gave way to a middle class identified by both their relation to capital as producers and consumers and a normal sexuality that leads to reproduction.[28]

The Gothic novel, I have been arguing, establishes the terms of monstrosity that were to be, and indeed were in the process of being, projected onto all who threatened the interests of a dwindling English nationalism. As the English empire stretched over oceans and continents, the need to define an essential English character became more and more pressing. Non-nationals, like Jews, for example, but also like the Irish or Gypsies, came to be increasingly identified by their alien natures and the concept of "foreign" became ever more closely associated with a kind of parasitical monstrosity, a non-reproductive sexuality, and an anti-English character. Gothic monsters in the 1880s and 1890s made parasitism — vampirism — the defining characteristic of horror. The parasitical nature of the beast might be quite literal, as in Stoker's vampire, or it might be a more indirect trait, as suggested by the creeping and homeless Hyde; it might be defined by a homoerotic influence, as exerted by Dorian Gray. Parasitism, especially with regards to the vampire, represents a bad or pathological sexuality, non-reproductive sexuality, a sexuality that exhausts and wastes and exists prior to and outside of the marriage contract.

The ability of race ideology and sexology to create a new elite to replace the aristocracy also allows for the staging of historical battles within the body. This suggests how Gothic monstrosity may intersect with, participate in, and resist the production of a theory of racial superiority. The Gothic monster—Frankenstein's creature, Hyde, Dorian Gray, and Dracula—represents the dramatization of the race question and of sexology in their many different incarnations. If Frankenstein's monster articulates the injustice of demonizing one's own productions, Hyde suggests that the most respectable bodies may be contaminated by bad blood; and if Dorian Gray's portrait makes an essential connection between the homosexual and the uncanny, Dracula embodies once and for all the danger of the hybrid race and the perverse sexuality within the form of the vampire.

The Power of Horror

In Gothic, as in many areas of Victorian culture, sexual material was not repressed but produced on a massive scale, as Michel Foucault has argued.[29] The narrative, then, that professed outrage at acts of sexual perversion (the nightly wanderings of Hyde, for example, or Dracula's midnight feasts) in fact produced a catalogue of perverse sexuality by first showcasing the temptations of the flesh in glorious technicolor and then by depicting so-called normal sex as a sickly enterprise devoid of all passion. One has only to think of the contrast between Mina Harker's encounter with Count Dracula—she is found lapping at blood from his breast—and her sexually neutral, maternal relations with her husband.

The production of sexuality as identity and as the inversion of identity (perversion—a turning away from identity) in Gothic novels consolidates normal sexuality by defining it in contrast to its monstrous manifestations. Horror, I have suggested, exercises power even as it incites pleasure and/or disgust. Horror, indeed, has a power closely related to its pleasure-producing function and the twin mechanism of pleasure-power perhaps explains how it is that Gothic may empower some readers even as it disables others. An example of how Gothic appeals differently to different readers may be found in contemporary slasher movies like *The Texas Chainsaw Massacre* (1974) and *Halloween*

(1978). Critics generally argue that these films inspire potency in a male viewer and incredible vulnerability in a female viewer. However, as we shall see in the later chapters of this book, the mechanisms of Gothic narrative never turn so neatly around gender identifications. A male viewer of the slasher film, like a male reader of the nineteenth-century Gothic, may find himself on the receiving end of countless acts of degradation in relation to monstrosity and its powers while the female reader and spectator may be able to access a surprising source of power through monstrous forms and monstrous genres.

In her psychoanalytic study of fear, *Powers of Horror,* Julia Kristeva defines horror in terms of "abjection." The abject, she writes, is "something rejected from which one does not part, from which one does not protect oneself as from an object. Imaginary uncanniness and real threat, it beckons to us and ends up engulfing us."[30] In a chapter on the writings of Celine, Kristeva goes on to identify abjection with the Jew of anti-Semitic discourse. Anti-Semitic fantasy, she suggests, elevates Jewishness to both mastery and weakness, to "sex tinged with femininity and death" (185).

The Jew, for Kristeva, anchors abjection within a body, a foreign body that retains a certain familiarity and that therefore confuses the boundary between self and other. The connection that Kristeva makes between psychological categories and socio-political processes leads her to claim that anti-Semitism functions as a receptacle for all kinds of fears — sexual, political, national, cultural, economic. This insight is important to the kinds of arguments that I am making about the economic function of the Gothic monster. The Jew in general within anti-Semitism is gothicized or transformed into a figure of almost universal loathing who haunts the community and represents its worst fears. By making the Jew supernatural, Gothic anti-Semitism actually makes Jews into spooks and Jew-hating into a psychological inevitability. The power of literary horror, indeed, lies in its ability to transform political struggles into psychological conditions and then to blur the distinction between the two. Literary horror, or Gothic, I suggest, uses the language of race hatred (most obviously anti-Semitism) to characterize monstrosity as a representation of psychological disorder. To understand the way monster may be equated with Jew or foreigner or non-English national, we need to historicize Gothic metaphors like vampire and parasite. We also have to read the effacement of the connection between monster and foreigner alongside the articulation of monster as a sexual category.

The Return of the Repressed

In an introduction to *Studies on Hysteria* written in 1893, Freud identifies the repressed itself as a foreign body. Noting that hysterical symptoms replay some original trauma in response to an accident, Freud explains that the memory of trauma "acts like a foreign body which, long after its entry, must continue to be regarded as an agent that is still at work."[31] In other words, until an original site of trauma reveals itself in therapy, it remains foreign to body and mind but active in both. The repressed, then, figures as a sexual secret that the body keeps from itself and it figures as foreign because what disturbs the body goes unrecognized by the mind.

The fiction that Freud tells about the foreign body as the repressed connects remarkably with the fiction Gothic tells about monsters as foreigners. Texts, like bodies, store up memories of past fears, of distant traumas. "Hysterics," writes Freud, "suffer mainly from reminiscences" (7). History, personal and social, haunts hysterics and the repressed always takes on an uncanny life of its own. Freud here has described the landscape of his own science — foreignness is repressed into the depths of an unconscious, a kind of cesspool of forgotten memories, and it rises to the surface as a sexual disturbance. Psychoanalysis gothicizes sexuality; that is to say, it creates a body haunted by a monstrous sexuality and forced into repressing its Gothic secrets. Psychoanalysis, in the Freudian scenario, is a sexual science able to account for and perhaps cure Gothic sexualities. Gothicization in this formula, then, is the identification of bodies in terms of what they are not. A Gothic other stabilizes sameness, a gothicized body is one that disrupts the surface-depth relationship between the body and the mind. It is the body that must be spoken, identified, or eliminated.

Eve Sedgwick has advanced a reading of Gothic as the return of the repressed. She reads fear in the Gothic in terms of the trope of "live burial" and finds in Gothic "a carceral sublime of representation, of the body, and potentially of politics and history as well" (*Coherence,* vi). Live burial as a trope is, of course, standard fare in the Gothic, particularly in eighteenth-century Gothic like Matthew Lewis's *The Monk* and Ann Radcliffe's *The Mysteries of Udolpho.* Live burial also works nicely as a metaphor for a repressed thing that threatens to return. Sedgwick's example of the repressed in Gothic is homosexuality. She characterizes the "paranoid Gothic novel" in terms of its thematization of homophobia and thus, she describes *Frankenstein*'s plot in terms of "a tableau of two men chasing each other across the landscape" (*Coherence,* ix).

But Sedgwick's reading tells only half the story. The sexual outsider in Gothic, I am suggesting, is always also a racial pariah, a national outcast, a class outlaw. The "carceral sublime of representation" that, for Sedgwick, marks the role of textuality or language in the production of fear does not only symbolize that Gothic language buries fear alive. Live burial is certainly a major and standard trope of Gothic but I want to read it alongside the trope of parasitism. Parasitism, I think, adds an economic dimension to live burial that reveals the entanglement of capital, nation, and the body in the fictions of otherness sanctified and popularized by any given culture. If live burial, for Sedgwick, reveals a "queerness of meaning," an essential doubleness within language that plays itself out through homoerotic doubles within the text, the carceral in my reading hinges upon a more clearly metonymic structure. Live burial as parasitism, then, becomes a tooth buried in an exposed neck for the explicit purpose of blood sucking or a monstrous Hyde hidden within the very flesh of a respectable Jekyll. Live burial is the entanglement of self and other within monstrosity and the parasitical relationship between the two. The one is always buried in the other.

The form of the Gothic novel, again as Sedgwick remarks, reflects further upon the parasitical monstrosity it creates. The story buried within a story buried within a story that Shelley's *Frankenstein* popularizes evolves into the narrative with one story but many different tellers. This form is really established by Wilkie Collins's *The Woman in White* (1860). In this novel, Collins uses a series of narrators so that almost every character in the novel tells his or her side of the story. Such a narrative device gives the effect of completion and operates according to a kind of judicial model of narration where all witnesses step forward to give an account. Within this narrative system, the author professes to be no more than a collector of documents, a compiler of the facts of the case. The reader, of course, is the judge and jury, the courtroom audience, and often, a kind of prosecuting presence expected to know truth, recognize guilt, and penalize monstrosity.

In *Dracula* Bram Stoker directly copies Collins's style. Stevenson also uses Collins's narrative technique in *Dr. Jekyll and Mr. Hyde* but he frames his story in a more overtly legal setting so that our main narrator is a lawyer, the central document is the last will and testament of Dr. Jekyll, and all other accounts contribute to the "strange case." All Gothic novels employing this narrative device share an almost obsessive concern with documentation and they all exhibit a sinister mistrust of the not-said, the unspoken, the hidden, and the silent. Furthermore, most Gothic novels lack the point of view of the monster. Collins does include in his novel a chapter by the notorious Count Fosco but Fosco's account is written as a forced confession that confirms his guilt and reveals his machinations. Neither Dracula nor Dorian Gray ever directly give their versions of events and Jekyll stands in at all times for his monstrous double, Hyde.

Collins's novel is extremely important to the Victorian Gothic tradition in that it establishes a layered narrative structure in which a story must be peeled back to reveal the secret or repressed center. The secret buried in the heart of Gothic, I suggested much earlier, is usually identified as a sexual secret. In an essay on the function of sensationalism in *The Woman in White*, Ann Cvetkovich argues that the sexual secret in this novel ultimately has little to do with a random sexual desire and everything to do with the class structure that brings Walter Hartright into contact with his future bride, Laura Fairlie. Cvetkovich suggests that the novel, in fact, sensationalizes class relations by making the relationship between Laura and her lowly art teacher seem fateful—preordained rather than a product of one man's social ambition.[32]

Novels in a Gothic mode transform class and race, sexual and national relations into supernatural or monstrous features. The threat posed by the Gothic monster is a combination of money, science, perversion, and imperialism but by reducing it to solely sexual aberrance, we fail to historicize Gothic embodiments.

The Technology of Monsters

This book will argue that Gothic novels are technologies that produce the monster as a remarkably mobile, permeable, and infinitely interpretable body. The monster's body, indeed, is a machine that, in its Gothic mode, produces meaning and can represent any horrible trait that the reader feeds into the narrative. The monster functions as monster, in other words, when it is able to condense as many fear-producing traits as possible into one body. Hence the sense that Frankenstein's monster is bursting out of his skin—he is indeed filled to bursting point with flesh and meaning both. Dracula, at the other end of the nineteenth century, is a body that consumes to excess—the vampiric body in its ideal state is a bloated body, sated with the blood of its victims.

Monsters are meaning machines. They can represent gender, race,

nationality, class, and sexuality in one body. And even within these divisions of identity, the monster can still be broken down. Dracula, for
example, can be read as aristocrat, a symbol of the masses; he is predator
and yet feminine, he is consumer and producer, he is parasite and host,
he is homosexual and heterosexual, he is even a lesbian. Monsters and
the Gothic fiction that creates them are therefore technologies, narrative
technologies that produce the perfect figure for negative identity. Monsters have to be everything the human is not and, in producing the
negative of human, these novels make way for the invention of human as
white, male, middle class, and heterosexual.

But Gothic is also a narrative technique, a generic spin that transforms the lovely and the beautiful into the abhorrent and then frames
this transformation within a humanist moral fable. A brilliant postmodern example of what happens when a narrative is gothicized is Tim
Burton's surrealistic *Nightmare Before Christmas* (1993). *Nightmare* is
an animated fantasy about what happens when Halloween takes over
Christmas. Halloween and Christmas, in this film, are conceived as
places rather than times or occasions and they each are embodied by
their festive representatives, Jack Skeleton and Santa Claus. Indeed religious or superstitious meanings of these holidays are almost entirely
absent from the plot. Jack Skeleton is a kind of melancholic romantic
hero who languishes under the strain of representing fear and maintain-
ing the machinery of horror every year. He stumbles upon the place
called Christmas one day after a stroll through the woods beyond his
graveyard and he decides that he wants to do Christmas this year instead
of Halloween.

The transformation of Christmas into Halloween is the gothicization of the sentimental; presents and toys, food and decorations are all
transformed from cheery icons of goodwill into fanged monsters, death
masks, and all manner of skullduggery. Kids are frightened, parents are
shocked, Santa Claus is kidnapped, and mayhem ensues. Of course, a
pathetic sentimental heroine called Sally uses her rag-doll body to restore
law and order and to woo Jack back to his proper place but nonetheless,
the damage has been done. Christmas, the myth of a transcendent gener-
osity, goodwill, and community love has been unmasked as just another
consumer ritual and its icons have been exposed as simply toys without
teeth or masks that smile instead of grimace. The naturalness and good-
ness of Christmas has unraveled and shown itself to be the easy target of
any and all attempts to make it Gothic.

While *Nightmare* suggests that, at least in a postmodern setting, gothicization seems to have progressive and even radicalizing effects, it is not always so simple to tell whether the presence of Gothic registers a conservative or a progressive move. Of course, Gothic is, as I have been arguing, mobile and therefore, we should not expect it to succumb so easily to attempts to make a claim for its political investments. But it does seem as if there has been a transformation in the uses of Gothic from the early nineteenth century to the present. The second part of my study attempts to read the contemporary horror film in order to argue that horror now disrupts dominant culture's representations of family, heterosexuality, ethnicity, and class politics. It disrupts, furthermore, the logic of genre that essentializes generic categories and stabilizes the production of meaning within them. Gothic film horror, I propose, produces models of reading (many in any one location) that allow for multiple interpretations and a plurality of locations of cultural resistance.

In this study I am using terms like "Gothic" and "technology" very specifically. Gothic has typically been used to refer to two sets of novels: first, to refer to Gothic revival novels of the late eighteenth century and then second, to refer to a cluster of fin-de-siècle novels in England. Obviously this study is more concerned with the latter group but I am not simply using Gothic as a generic organizing term. Gothic, I will be arguing, is the breakdown of genre and the crisis occasioned by the inability to "tell," meaning both the inability to narrate and the inability to categorize. Gothic, I argue, marks a peculiarly modern preoccupation with boundaries and their collapse. Gothic monsters, furthermore, differ from the monsters that come before the nineteenth century in that the monsters of modernity are characterized by their proximity to humans.

This book follows Gothic monstrosity through its various incarnations in fiction and film and across two centuries. In chapter 2, "Making Monsters: Mary Shelley's *Frankenstein*," I read *Frankenstein* as an allegory of the history of the novel. Mary Shelley, I argue, produces a "totalizing" monster who defines the cultural and symbolic functions of monstrosity. This monster signifies an array of societal, political, and sexual threats and must be read as a textual technology and a Gothic history of narrative itself. In the next chapter, on *The Strange Case of Dr. Jekyll and Mr. Hyde* and *The Picture of Dorian Gray,* I examine these two Gothic texts as inversions of each other which both produce a model of human subjectivity predicated on a topology of surface and depth. Hyde is hidden within Jekyll and Dorian Gray's picture takes upon its own surface the traces of his debauched life. In each case inner and outer identities are layered over each other to produce the effects of humanity, perversity, racial impurity, and degeneration. My fourth chapter, on Bram Stoker's *Dracula,* understands *Dracula* to be a cornerstone of Gothic writing in that it produces another "totalizing" monster, a brother to Frankenstein's monster, who represents the fate of anarchic consumption. In my reading of the vampire's particular brand of monstrosity, I comment upon the peculiar consistencies between the Gothic vampire and the anti-Semite's Jew.

The second half of *Skin Shows* begins to trace Gothic monstrosity into the twentieth century and into contemporary horror film. I use psychoanalysis in chapter 5 in order to bridge the gap between nineteenth- and twentieth-century conceptions of monstrosity, fear, and horror. In keeping with my claim throughout that fear and monstrosity are historically specific forms rather than psychological universals, I try to account for a switch in emphasis within the representation and interpretation of monstrous bodies from class, race, and nationality to a primary focus upon sexuality and gender. In large part, this narrowing down of monstrous features to monstrous sex and gender has to do with the success of the hegemonic installation of psychoanalytic interpretations of human subjectivity which understand subjectivity as sexual subjectivity and identity as sexual identity and monstrosity as sexual pathology. Freud's case histories of paranoia illustrate well the psychoanalytic fictions of fear and loathing which tend to revolve around a rather homophobic insistence on paranoia as fear of homosexual desire. I conclude this chapter by reading Freud's case of paranoia in a woman against the grain and arguing for a productive site of inquiry into fear through female paranoia that may produce feminist readings of horror.

To demonstrate the effects of a psychoanalytic account of horror and fear, I graft my analysis of Freud's case history of paranoia in a woman onto Alfred Hitchcock's *The Birds* (1963). It becomes clear immediately that the cinematic monstrosity of the birds represents something very different, and functions differently, than the textual horror of Frankenstein's monster and Dracula. As we will see in relation to postmodern horror film, the postmodern era does not offer any totalizing monsters, and meaning refuses to coalesce within one hideous body. The birds themselves in Hitchcock's film are a good example of the transference of horror from a specifically unnatural body to nature itself embodied within the myriad form of a flock of aggressive birds. The horror genre itself, as it moves from book to cinema, from word to image shatters into many pieces and every horror film simultaneously creates the genre anew and conforms loosely to the conventions of a subgenre.

In order to trace the evolution of a post-psychoanalytic cinema of cruelty, I examine symptomatic instances within two models of horror. While one's first impulse might be to mark these models as "masculine" and "feminine," gender soon becomes inadequate as an axis of identification. While a film like *The Birds* seems to readily offer itself to a psychoanalytic interpretation based upon gender identifications, a later subgenre known as "splatter cinema" seems to refuse the neat classification of aberrant gender horror. Splatter films themselves have a long history going back to the early Hammer films based upon the myths of Frankenstein and Dracula and it is this genre which seems to continue the Gothic lineage of the nineteenth-century Gothic novel. Even in relation to the avowed economic motivation behind the production of Gothic, Hammer films and nineteenth-century Gothic are in accord. Sir James Carrera, the founder and president of Hammer film productions, is quoted as saying, "We're in the business to make money, not to win Oscars. If the public were to decide tomorrow that it wanted Strauss waltzes, we'd be in the Strauss waltz business."[33] It is not hard to hear in this statement an echo of Robert Louis Stevenson's justification of his "Gothic gnome." Also implicit in Carreras's words is the connection between monstrous art, monstrous economy, and the perverse pleasures of the public.

Horror, in other words, within twentieth-century cinema has both a high-culture and a low-culture life. *The Birds,* of course, belongs to the oeuvre of auteur Alfred Hitchcock while much splatter horror is made by low-budget gore masters. The mind/body split that divides nineteenth-century Gothic from nineteenth-century realism is reproduced here as the difference between films for money that depict graphic violence for a voyeuristic audience and films for art's sake which depict the epic struggles of human against other. And popularity is not the difference between these two branches of Gothic cinema; the difference again lies in the depiction of bodily monstrosity and the division of fear into psychological and physiological categories. Nowadays, of course, the psychological horror film is called the "thriller" and in the psychoanalytic tradition, it tends to represent fear through narratives about rape and sexual murder (*Jagged Edge, Unlawful Entry, Blink*).

Since I do not have room in this study to catalogue the horror genre in any kind of comprehensive manner, I examine representative films from high and low Gothic cinema in order to give a symptomatic history of the horror film and to show how it descends from nineteenth-century Gothic. I look first at Hitchcock's *The Birds* as an example of female paranoia which bears comparison to Freud's case history of a paranoid woman and as an example of the psychohorror lodged within the heart of the ordinary, the natural, and the everyday. Next, I turn to a lugubrious example of splatter cinema in *The Texas Chainsaw Massacre 2*.

My final chapter, on *The Silence of the Lambs,* claims that this film is important to the genre partly because it represents the horror of the extraordinary and the horror of the ordinary side by side but also because it marks the place where low-budget basement gore comes to mainstream Hollywood as an art film. It is not enough to remark that Jonathan Demme, therefore, sells out the cult status of the B movie and transforms it into a mainstream commodity, rather Demme robs liberally from both the psychodrama and the blood fest to create the thinking person's splatter film. Demme's later work, like the deplorable *Philadelphia* (1994), suggests what makes him so suited for this function of cleaning up the splatter genre—he is part of a new crop of blockbuster directors, including Oliver Stone and Steven Spielburg, who manage to capitalize on the popularity of a subject without acknowledging any of the material conditions which make that subject popular.

Throughout my readings of the horror film, I stress the role of reception and call for a Gothic spectatorship, a set of practices not bound by the strict rules of psychoanalytic film theory. I suggest the limits of psychoanalytic readings of horror and I call simultaneously for feminist and queer Gothic readings. Since the horror film, as I have suggested, seems to locate monstrosity primarily within monstrous gender and monstrous sexuality and since the predations of the monster inevitably focus upon a female victim, feminist and queer responses to these Gothic modalities are most certainly called for if we are to make a claim for the positivity of horror. Any consideration of monstrosity within contemporary film, in other words, has to reckon with the function of male violence and female passivity. I suggest that we apply the insights learned from nineteenth-century Gothic to twentieth-century Gothic to read the monster as mobile and open to multiple interpretations and the Gothic text itself as a meaning machine available for any number of readings.

In my final two chapters, then, I attempt extended readings of some of the different trajectories of Gothic monstrosity within the modern slasher film. In the chapters on *The Texas Chainsaw Massacre 2* and *The*

Silence of the Lambs, I argue that they reproduce the terms, conditions, and technologies of nineteenth-century Gothic horror but tend to shift the position of monstrosity within those narratives. The monster, eventually, is no longer totalizing. The monstrous body that once represented everything is now represented as potentially meaning anything — it may be the outcast, the outlaw, the parasite, the pervert, the embodiment of uncontrollable sexual and violent urges, the foreigner, the misfit. The monster is all of these but monstrosity has become a conspiracy of bodies rather than a singular form. Milton, Blake once commented in relation to *Paradise Lost,* was of the devil's party. Within postmodern Gothic we are all of the devil's party. My final chapter, on *The Silence of the Lambs,* claims that monstrosity is almost a queer category that defines the subject as at least partially monstrous. Within postmodern Gothic we no longer attempt to identify the monster and fix the terms of his/her deformity, rather postmodern Gothic warns us to be suspicious of monster hunters, monster makers, and above all, discourses invested in purity and innocence. The monster always represents the disruption of categories, the destruction of boundaries, and the presence of impurities and so we need monsters and we need to recognize and celebrate our own monstrosities.

2

Making Monsters:

Mary Shelley's Frankenstein

Monster Making

When Victor Frankenstein animates the lump of flesh and skin and bones that he has assembled in his "filthy workshop of creation," he brings to life body horror. While the Gothic Romances of the 1790s associated horror with locale, Frankenstein's monster makes flesh itself Gothic and Shelley, therefore, maps out a new geography of terror and finds fear to be a by-product of embodiment rather than a trick played upon the body by the mind. Although *Frankenstein* is not always classified as a Gothic novel (it is often identified as science fiction), I begin my history of Gothic with this novel because of its preoccupation with bodily monstrosity and because, in some senses, the story of the conflict between Frankenstein and his monster, an author and his creation, resonates with the history of the novel itself.

The importance of Mary Shelley's *Frankenstein* (1816) within the Gothic tradition, modern mythology, the history of the novel, and a cultural history of fear and prejudice cannot be emphasized too strongly. *Frankenstein* not only gives form to the dialectic of monstrosity itself and raises questions about the pleasures and dangers of textual production, it also demands a rethinking of the entire Gothic genre in terms of *who* rather than *what* is the object of terror. By focusing upon the body as the locus of fear, Shelley's novel suggests that it is people (or at least bodies) who terrify people, not ghosts or gods, devils or monks, windswept castles or labyrinthine monasteries. The architecture of fear in this story is replaced by physiognomy, the landscape of fear is replaced by sutured skin, the conniving villain is replaced by an antihero and his monstrous creation, and the antihero as well as his offspring are both writers and readers. Meanwhile, the heroine, who in the Gothic Romance was transported from one prisonlike structure to another, is now a metaphor for the domestic prison that threatens to entrap Frankenstein and keep him from his solitary, Faust-like enterprise. She is also metonymically linked to the monster, however, since the grotesqueries of the human form are linked, in this novel, to an extreme fear of feminine sexual response.[1]

Frankenstein's monster has attained mythic status within both the popular imagination and the critical project of literary history. Exhaustive studies of *Frankenstein* have read the monster's symbolic value in terms of sex, gender, and class. The monster, in various readings then, is literature, women's creativity, Mary Shelley herself; the monster is class struggle, the product of industrialization, a representation of the proletariat; the monster is all social struggle, a specific symbol of the French Revolution, the power of the masses unleashed; the monster is technology, the danger of science without conscience, the autonomous machine. As Franco Moretti so aptly states, like Dracula, Frankenstein's creature is a "totalizing monster"[2] — one, in other words, who threatens to never be vanquished, one immune to temporary restorations of order and peace. Totalizing, of course, does not mean essential. Essential monstrosity makes monstrosity an integral feature of very specific bodies; totalized monstrosity allows for a whole range of specific monstrosities to coalesce in the same form.

The "totalizing monster," a modern invention, threatens community from all sides and from its very core rather than from a simple outside. The chameleonic nature of this monster makes it a symbol of multiplicity and indeed invites multiple interpretations. One critic, Marie-Helene Huet, in *The Monstrous Imagination,* has made the obvious but necessary connection between monstrosity and prodigious generativity. Huet argues that monstrosity within Romanticism tells of "the dark desire to reproduce without the other" and represents art as the resulting progeny of unnatural reproduction.[3] In general, however, various critics have attempted to narrow the scope of monstrosity in *Frankenstein* in order to theorize fear and a semiotic of horror. Such critical accounts tend to exclude or de-emphasize the monster's status as hybrid in favor of specific class- or gender-inflected readings. In any attempt to fix monstrosity, some aspect of it escapes unread. Moretti, for example, having named the monster as "totalizing," also makes a strong case for the monster as the proletariat, "a collective and artificial creature" (85). Describing Frankenstein himself as the bourgeois subject conscious of "having produced his own grave-diggers" (86), Moretti goes on to suggest that Frankenstein and his monster are unable to play out their proper roles as owner and worker because, for Shelley, "the demands of production have no value in themselves, but must be subordinated to the maintenance of the moral and material solidity of the family" (90).

Moretti understands the technology of the monster narrative to be one which subordinates class to family but in fact it is crucial to recognize that monsters play precisely upon the boundaries that seem to neatly delineate family from class, personal from economic, sexual from political. Owner and worker relations, in other words, are precisely played out in family relations; the narrative of family is indeed the sentimentalized version, or in this case the gothicized version, of class struggle and race war. Shelley's *Frankenstein* confirms, in fact, that the construction of the monster facilitates rather than emanates from the construction of "the family." The family, indeed, in this novel, is as fragmented and incoherent as the monster himself and it only takes on a glow of authenticity in the absence of all family members. Hence, at the outermost frame of the novel we have a reader, Mrs. Saville, Walton's sister, a married woman who rests comfortably at home in England. Mrs. Saville represents the way that home and family exist as imaginary limits to the narratives of voyage and discovery. At the innermost frame of the novel, of course, we have a picture-perfect family but the family in question represents domestic bliss as the union of a European man (Felix) and his subjugated Oriental bride (Safie). As Joseph W. Lew comments in an article, "The Deceptive Other: Mary Shelley's Critique of Orientalism in *Frankenstein*," this family represents itself as the safe haven of the Oriental woman from the barbarity of the East.[4]

When Moretti does touch briefly upon the fact that the monster of class may also be representative of other forms of monstrosity, he seems unable to recognize the full significance of the potentiality of any one form of othering to become another. He remarks upon Frankenstein's fear that his monster, if given a mate, will bring a "race of devils" into the world; Mary Shelley, according to Moretti, at her most reactionary, turns the class other, the proletariat, into a "race of devils" and so, he claims, she transforms a historical product into a "natural" and immutable category. But Moretti has also transformed one category into another here; he has assigned class to the order of the artificial and he has naturalized race. A reading of Gothic monstrosity attuned to the specific technology of monsters demands that identity itself be read as a constructed category, one that depends heavily upon the mutual and interdependent constructions of race, class, and gender.[5]

The very project of interpretation in this novel, I am saying, is complex and unstable and it is this instability, in part, that generates the infinite interpretability of the monster. As Daniel Cottom writes: "Frankenstein's monster images the monstrous nature of representation."[6] The monster defies definition just as the novel itself seems to challenge neat generic categories. The question, What is it? in other words, has to be directed both at the book and the monster. Indeed, the connection between the two is made perfectly clear by Mary Shelley in her introduction when she dubs her book "my hideous progeny" and bids it "go forth and prosper." The question that haunts the monster, Who am I? is repeated in critical gestures toward the novel that ask, What is it? The answer, of course, lies in the impossibility of pinning definition to this peculiar form.

The form of the novel is its monstrosity; its form opens out onto excess because, like the monster of the story, the sum of the novel's parts exceeds the whole. Its structure, the exoskeleton, and not its dignified contents — philosophies of life, meditations on the sublime, sentimental narratives of family and morality, discussions of aesthetics — makes this novel a monster text. The monstrosity of *Frankenstein* is literally built into the textuality of the novel to the point where textual production itself is responsible for generating monsters.

Because definition is beside the point, then, the questions to direct at the monstrous book are (1) what exactly constitutes its productivity?, (2) how does it reproduce within the domain of interpretation?, and (3) are we, the readers, the "race of devils" that Frankenstein feared he would loose upon the world? I want to answer these questions by looking closely at the narrative form of the novel and then by suggesting that possibly the novel plays out an allegory of Gothic fiction itself, or that the Gothic plays out an allegory of the production of the novel. There are, of course, in this text, two monsters that Frankenstein attempts to bring to life, one male and one female. The aborted female monster can be read as the ugly popular fiction, Gothic fiction, that is always debased in relation to some notion of high culture. She is the body of work that is always "half-finished," that inspires violence, and that literally is reduced to pulp. This relationship between popularity and population (since the female monster represents precisely Frankenstein's fear of a monstrous reproduction) needs to be thought through in relation to recent histories of the novel and to the main narrative of human versus monster that Frankenstein and his creation enact.

I suggest that the book presents itself not as the making of a monster but as the making of a human. In what ways does the monster construct Frankenstein, in other words? Who actually builds whom and who destroys whom? The construction of the human will frame my discussion of monstrosity throughout this book and in relation to this novel, I am concerned to link the construction of humanness to a split within the novel between popular and high culture but also to the dependent histories of race, nation, gender, and sexuality. The identity of a Frankenstein, in other words, always depends utterly upon the various lines of constructions that coalesce in his humanity. His humanness depends as much upon his status as male, bourgeois, and white as the monster's monstrosity depends upon his yellow skin, his gargantuan size, his masslike shape, and his unstable gender. First, however, let's look at the machinery, the textual machine, that generates meaning in *Frankenstein*.

Monstrous Forms

The framing device which structures *Frankenstein* skews perspective and complicates relations between author and narrator, author and readers, and between characters. The novel's first frame (although "first" is a contested notion in this novel, and this frame is already preceded by the author's introductions and an epigraph from Milton's *Paradise Lost*) is a series of letters from Walton to his sister, Margaret Saville (whose initials, M.S., of course, suggest the conflation of author, Mary Shelley; and reader, Margaret Saville; and manuscript). Next, we read in Walton's journal of his meeting with Victor and his transcription of Victor's story. Within Victor's story we read letters from Elizabeth and then the monster's story. The monster recounts his discovery of Victor's journal within his description of how he came to know himself as monstrous and human in his time spent with the De Laceys. We return finally to Walton's ship, the *Archangel*, to Victor's deathbed. Victor dies and the monster disappears into the darkness.

Frankenstein generates stories and narrative perspectives like a machine. Chris Baldick's study, *In Frankenstein's Shadow,* contrasts the construction of the monster from fragments of corpses to the structure of the novel as an aggregate of narrative pieces and furthermore, to the absorption and reproduction by Mary Shelley of a mass of literary influences from Milton to the writings of her mother and father. Baldick suggests that "there is a fund of literary sources upon which *Frankenstein* cannibalistically feeds."[7] Baldick's notion of cannibalistic activity is, I think, extremely important to both *Frankenstein* and the Gothic genre in general. Bram Stoker's *Dracula* also functions according to a model of consumption and production; it too assembles a writing machine from letters and journals, dictaphones and phonographs; it too feeds cannibalistically on its sources. The structures of both *Frankenstein* and *Dracula* activate and exemplify models of production and consumption which suggest that Gothic, as a genre, is itself a hybrid form, a stitched body of distorted textuality. This model also has obvious links to the capitalist structures that produced the novel as a commodity which brought income to writers and was paid for by (mostly middle-class) readers.

In order to explain the cannibalistic activity that I think is associated with Gothic form, I want to link Baldick's comment about *Frankenstein*'s cannibalistic activity to a theory advanced by Nancy Armstrong in *Desire and Domestic Fiction* of the "omnivorous behavior" of the novel. I quote:

> [I]f, as I believe is the case, the novel contains the history of sexuality within it, then its own history — the history of fiction — is displaced along with that "other" history. Given the omnivorous behavior I am attributing to the novel, there is very little cultural material that cannot be included within the feminine domain. Consequently there is very little political information that cannot be transformed into psychological information.[8]

Armstrong shows how "omnivorous behavior" in the novel means that domestic fiction participates in, rather than represents, the production of female subjects. Furthermore, by transforming political identities into sexual identities, political resistance is diffused by the novel and "the feminine domain" remains in bondage to a metaphysics of gender.

Gothic, I suggest, beginning with *Frankenstein,* is a textual machine, a technology that transforms class struggle, hostility towards women, and tensions arising out of the emergent ideology of racism into what look like sexual or psychosexual battles between and within individuals. The monster is consistently read as his maker's alter ego, as his unconscious, as the return of the repressed. Moretti, who otherwise concentrates on the materialist dimensions of the monster, claims that this figure cannot be adequately explained by recourse to economic or historical terms and he suggests that the monster is "the rhetorical figure" that both "expresses the unconscious content and at the same time hides it" (103). The monster as metaphor, still according to Moretti, transforms social and psychic fears ("the fear of monopoly capital and the fear of the mother") into other forms "so that readers do not have to face up to what really frightens them" (105).

Moretti's marxist-based notion that monsters allow for the expansion and enrichment "of the structures of false consciousness" differs significantly from the kind of transformation that I am noting in terms of Gothic technologies. Monsters, like the one Frankenstein builds, embody a multiplicity of fears and invite the reader to participate in charting the shapes and contours of each one. Most often, the postpsychoanalytic modern reader assumes that Gothic monstrosity occupies a privileged relation to a psychology of horror but this assumes the transhistorical availability of psychic interpretations and understandings of the self. The reason we can read the monster as a psychic structure is because the monster can take the imprint of that interpretation not because that interpretation most usefully describes monstrosity. Monsters appeal to readers and consumers because they represent in their very form the game of reading and writing, rewriting and telling, telling and interpreting. False consciousness is simply not an issue here because no reading is false. The cannibalism of the Gothic form, its consumption of its own sources, allows for the infinitude of interpretation because each fear, each literary source, each desire, each historical event, each social structure that the text preys upon becomes fuel for the manufacture of meanings.

Frankenstein's monster in particular, since he is given a voice, complicates the cannibalistic narrative structure by participating in it even as he is revealed as a product and a symbol of that structure. The narrative frames, furthermore, allow us to trace the transformations that take place in Gothic of racial, sexual, historical, and psychological into metaphoric, of productive into representative. Furthermore, the Gothic form is implicated in the monstrosity it produces because, as a mutation of classic realism, it is regarded as an ugly, clumsy, and fantastical genre. And the monster—like the "zoophagous" Renfield in *Dracula* who desires "to absorb as many lives as possible" by eating cats that have eaten mice that have eaten spiders that have eaten flies — the monster can be broken down into the lives and forms he has absorbed.

Eve Sedgwick's discussion of the trope of "live burial" has obvious significance to a theory of Gothic's cannibalistic nature. Sedgwick writes: "If the story-within-etc. represents the broadest structural application of the otherwise verbal or thematic convention of the unspeakable, it has a similar relation to the convention of live burial."[9] Sedgwick is interested in charting a topography of Gothic where a certain spatial relation pertains to the tropes of inside and outside, live burial, and the unspeakable in Gothic. Gothic, then, according to Sedgwick, is marked by a doubleness of space created violently by the destruction of boundaries. One space (inside, silence, nightmare) encroaches or feeds upon another (outside, speech, experience) as the difficulty of telling becomes a part of the act of confession. Ultimately, for Sedgwick, language performs the operations of the uncanny so that the unspeakable is buried alive within the speakable, one story lies buried in another, one history produces and buries others.

In *Frankenstein* it is identity itself which is buried alive, or rather which is figured as live burial. The epigraph to the novel, Adam's question to God in book 10 of *Paradise Lost,* "Did I request thee, Maker, from my Clay/To mould me Man?" already conceives of the human as something that has been built, in this instance by God from clay. Obviously, the relationship between Victor Frankenstein and his monster parodies the relationship between God and Adam/Satan/Eve but it also replaces a divine relation with a secular one. The epigraph sets *Frankenstein* up against the most authoritative creation myth in Western culture but it is crucial to note that the novel is not comparing itself to the creation story but rather to its literary recounting in Milton's epic poem. Origins, in *Frankenstein,* are always literary or textual rather than religious or scientific.

Furthermore, the question posed by the epigraph emphasizes the problem of definition — what is human? what is a human relationship? how do we recognize humanity? These become questions that this novel directs specifically at the problem of form. In this novel the monster is not human because he lacks the proper body — he is too big, too ugly, disproportionate. He is also a question directed at nature; Frankenstein had hoped to discover "nature's secrets" with his creation but his monster is no answer to nature's mysteries, so-called, he is simply another question. He is the body that produces the natural and the human as power relations and his is the body that uses up natural and human remains in order to recycle flesh into scientific invention.

By marking Gothic as cannibalistic, as an essentially consumptive genre which feeds parasitically upon other literary texts, I want to draw attention to the violence with which the form erases boundaries and consumes stories and lives in order to produce fear. The production of fear is, therefore, the result of a technology that simultaneously produces an epistemological crisis. The reading subject (but also the characters and seemingly the writer) of the Gothic is constructed out of a kind of paranoia about boundaries: Do I read or am I written? Am I monster or monster maker? Am I monster hunter or the hunted? Am I human or other? For the modern reader such questions might seem to circle around sexual identity, Who/what do I desire? But nineteenth-century monstrosity confounds the possibility of a single answer to the question of identity. If we read *Frankenstein* as a story about repressed homoerotic desire, for example, we risk not reading it as a story about childbirth; and if we only read it as a "birth myth," we miss the narrative of class.

Narrative resolution in Gothic fiction, of course, usually resolves boundary disputes by the end of the novel by killing off the monster and restoring law and order but fear lingers on because after all, in *Frankenstein* the monster as subject is produced through the reading of texts. The monster comes to knowledge, self-knowledge, by reading the books he finds at the De Laceys' and finding himself in his own drama of identification. After reading *Paradise Lost,* for example, he is compelled to ask whether he is another Adam "apparently united by no link to any other being in existence."[10] But, he concludes, "I considered Satan as the fitter emblem of my condition" (129). Feminist critics have also noted a remarkable resemblance between the monster and Eve.[11] Notice, however, that nothing is gained by fixing the monster to one of these identities. While the epigraph to Shelley's book suggests strongly that, in his drama of creation, the monster is indeed Adam, asking, like Adam, "Did I request thee, Maker, from my Clay / To mould me Man?" the feminist reading that identifies bodily monstrosity with a fear of femininity demands that the monster be stabilized as female; and the conventional reading that understands the monster as flawed humanity makes him into a kind of Satan figure.

The monster is always all of these figures. By his very composition, he can never be one thing, never represent only a singular anxiety. His formation out of bits and pieces of life and death, of criminals and animals, animate and inanimate objects means that he is always in danger of breaking down into his constitutive parts. It is the propensity for the monster to deconstruct at any time, to always be in the process of decomposition, that makes it/him/her a fugitive from identity and a model for the Gothic reader.

It is also a kind of ahistorical desire on the part of the modern reader that seeks an answer to the question of identity in the form of the monster. By demanding that the monster round out our definitions of "human" (either by representing a polar opposite or by showing "real humanity") we also remake the monster as alien, as other, as difference. The monster, in fact, is where we come to know ourselves as never-human, as always between humanness and monstrosity. Just as, for the monster, paradise is always lost in *Frankenstein,* so, for the reader, humanity — humane treatment of others, justice, etc. — is always beyond our reach.

After Justine has been killed for the death of William, Elizabeth mourns for her lost vision of the "human":

> "When I reflect my dear cousin," said she, "on the miserable death of Justine Moritz, I no longer see the world and its works as they before appeared to me. Before I looked upon the accounts of vice and injustice, that I read in books or heard from others, as tales of ancient days or imaginary evils; at least they were remote, and more familiar to reason than to the imagination; but now misery has come home, and men appear to me as monsters thirsting for each other's blood." (92–93)

This is a remarkable statement of an antisentimental view of human nature which is all the more powerful in that it comes from Elizabeth, the representative of family and community in the novel. Elizabeth very accurately describes how the human is a complicated structure that depends at least in part upon a vision of progress from past "vice and injustice" to present equity and humanity; she recognizes that "tales of . . . imaginary evils" construct a vision of false harmony within a present tense; and finally she acknowledges that "now misery has come home, and men appear to me as monsters." The bleeding of one category into another that we have noted as a feature of Gothic takes on a very significant function here. Elizabeth really gives us the key to Shelley's narrative in this speech. Monster seeps into the category of man as justice miscarries and misery comes home. It is the human that falls into doubt at this crucial moment; it is the human that seems to be a patchwork of morality, criminality, subterfuge, and domesticity, and one which barely holds together. Elizabeth, indeed, at crucial moments in the narrative fails to distinguish between man and monster and this becomes the new role of the heroine in Gothic. Where the heroine fails to distinguish, the distinction fails to hold. So, in *Dracula*, as we will see, Lucy and Mina are both seduced by the vampire and they fail to distinguish between his bite and the proper penetrations of their husbands and fiancés.

The production of the monster by Frankenstein throws humanness into relief because it emphasizes the constructedness of all identity. While superficially this novel seems to be about the making of a monster, it is really about the making of a human. It is also about the destruction of otherness, the unmaking of monstrosity that is demanded by the sentimental narrative of conquest, voyage, and discovery. Frankenstein's relationships with Clerval and Walton, his dependence upon other men for his own masculinity, means that he must repudiate both the monster's plea for empathy and the possibility of a female monster.

Visual Horror and Narrative

Beautiful! — Great God! His yellow skin scarcely covered the work of muscles and arteries beneath; his hair was of a lustrous black, and flowing; his teeth of a pearly whiteness; but these luxuriances only formed a more horrid contrast with his watery eyes, that seemed almost of the same colour as the dun white sockets in which they were set, his shrivelled complexion and straight black lips. (57)

Frankenstein's monster's skin barely covers his interior—the monster is transparent. The features that should make him beautiful, furthermore, "lustrous black" hair and "teeth of a pearly whiteness," look hideous because they are out of place in relation to the "watery eyes" and "shrivelled complexion." The monster is both skintight and "shrivelled," he has beautiful features set next to extreme ugliness. The whole impression is underscored by the "straight black lips"—evidence of a lack of internal circulation, evidence of the borrowed nature of all of his most necessary features. All in all, the monster is the obscenity of the surface, unwatchable, a masterpiece of a horror that cannot be viewed without terror.

It is no surprise that *Frankenstein* is the granddaddy of Gothic film horror. The horror film, after all, depends upon a certain degree of unwatchability. Cinematic horror also asks that the monster become a kind of screen onto which the spectator's fears are projected. In a way, *Frankenstein* establishes the preconditions for cinematic horror and for horror to become cinematic by making the monster's monstrosity so definitively visual. Only a blind man can accept the monster uncritically in this novel and, in a way, the blindness of old De Lacey represents also the blindness of the reader. We are disposed as readers to sympathize with the monster because, unlike the characters in the novel, we cannot see him. Once the monster becomes visible within contemporary horror films, monstrosity becomes less and less recuperable.

The monster in *Frankenstein* establishes visual horror as the main standard by which the monster judges and is judged. The most central episode in the novel, the narrative of the De Lacey family, establishes visual recognition as the most important code in the narrative of monstrosity. The story of the De Laceys is buried within the monster's story, their story is a subset of his, but his story (history) becomes a model of history itself as he learns of "the strange system of human society" and of "the division of property, of immense wealth and squalid poverty; of rank, descent, and noble blood" (120).

Just as the monster reads *Paradise Lost* as "a true history," so "true history" is reduced to the story of one family at the innermost recess of the novel. True history and fiction trade places so that the story of the family replaces the story of nations; and the narrative of the body replaces the history of creation; and the significance of visual codes becomes greater than that of heritage. The fiction of the monster replaces the history of discovery and invention that first Walton and then Frankenstein try to tell. And through these series of substitutions, the "true history" of the world boils down to the monster's reading list, a quirky canon of stories for underdogs, and a tale of subjectivity as a self-knowledge that inheres to the human.

But humanity as well as monstrosity, in this novel, depends upon visual codes for its construction. The women in Victor's family, Elizabeth, Caroline, and Justine, in their roles and fates in the novel, suggest the contradictions which lie at the heart of any attempt to distinguish definitively between human and monster. Elizabeth is rescued by Caroline from a peasant family. Caroline notices Elizabeth in the poor family's cottage because "she appeared of a different stock" (84). Elizabeth is "thin and very fair" while the peasant children are "dark-eyed, hardy little vagrants" (84). Indeed, it happens that Elizabeth is of "different stock" and the daughter of a nobleman, fit, therefore, for adoption. Caroline adopts Justine also but Justine must remain a servant since her heritage reveals no nobility. Birth, then, or blood rather, separates one woman from another and prepares one for marriage and the other for service. But notice that the difference between the noble and the debased is clearly exhibited in this instance upon the surface of the body — Elizabeth stands out from the rest of her poor family because she is thin and fair.

The class designation implied by "different stock," because it is a distinction based upon blood, exemplifies very well how, as Moretti suggests, "racial discrimination" springs from the narrative. Moretti, as we noted, finds racial discrimination in *Frankenstein* to be a way of transforming class into a natural and immutable category, but as the difference in status between Elizabeth and Justine shows, the transformation is more complicated than this. By emphasizing that Elizabeth stands out from the "dark-eyed, hardy little vagrants" in the peasant family, Shelley betrays a class-biased belief that not only is nobility inherent but aristocratic class coincides with aristocratic race and is therefore *visible*. Race discrimination, indeed, displaces or at least supplements class hierarchies in this narrative partly because the theme of visible monstrosity demands that identity be something that can be seen. The monster, as we know, represents the threat not of a new class but of a new *race* of beings.

The class gradations implied by the adoptions of Elizabeth as daughter and Justine as servant, then, hint at a tension within Shelley's writing between class, race, and gender. Both women are marked by their class (and class marking may be understood as race marking) in ways that make their Gothic fates inevitable. Elizabeth, as obviously middle class, must be sacrificed to the monster, and Justine, a lower-class servant, must stand in for the monster in the trial for the murder of William. On a certain level she doubles the female monster whose fate is always to be less than human. Configurations in the novel of class and gender, in fact, turn class into proletariat, gender into woman and oppose the two in relation to the monster. In other words, the only category that remains unmarked in the novel, the only category that seems "natural" is that of the bourgeois male and he, in the form of Victor and Walton, consequently comes to embody the human.

Visual codes by the end of the century in Gothic fiction came to signify predispositions for crime or sexual aberration. As we will see in

Stevenson's *Dr. Jekyll and Mr. Hyde* and Stoker's *Dracula,* bad bodies are easily identifiable and demand expulsion. But criminal anthropology of the 1890s also made essential connections between outward appearance and inward essence and it is here that we can discuss a ripple of Gothic form across a variety of scientific, cultural, and social narratives. While visual horror in *Frankenstein* is the reason that the monster must live his days in exile, in fin-de-siècle Gothic visual horror is the sign of a criminality that will demand expulsion. The difference between Frankensteinian horror and fin-de-siècle horror is, I will be arguing, a result of different conceptions of subjectivity. Gothic narratives in fiction, science, and social science combined to produce evil or criminality as a seed planted deep within an interior self. But how did the self come to be associated with interiority and how did truth come to be represented by a deep structure of subjectivity? One answer surely lies in the eruption of "sexuality" in the nineteenth century, a discourse and a technology which, as Foucault says, proliferates across disciplines. "The nineteenth century and our own," he writes, "have been rather the age of multiplication: a dispersion of sexualities, a strengthening of their disparate forms, a multiple implantation of 'perversions.' "[12]

While we have generally accepted Foucault's repudiation of the "repressive hypothesis" — of the claim, in other words, that Victorian culture repressed sexuality and replaced it with a highly regimented moral code — it has been less clear as to exactly how the production of sexualities came to look like repression. Also, how is it possible, as he claims, "to constitute a sexuality that is economically useful and politically conservative" and yet to make this constitutive process seem "natural"? The answer some theorists have come up with is, the novel. David Miller, for example, in *The Novel and the Police,* argues that the Victorian novel in its form and themes confirms "the novel-reader in his identity as 'liberal subject' " — as a subject, in other words, who considers him- or herself to be free. He writes: "Such confirmation is thoroughly imaginary, to be sure, but so too, I will eventually be suggesting, is the identity of the liberal subject, who seems to recognize himself most fully only when he forgets or disavows his functional implications in a system of carceral restraints or disciplinary injunctions."[13] The imaginary nature of the subject is closely related, therefore, to the subject's imagination; it is precisely when reading, when engaging with fictional realities, that we consider ourselves removed from the hustle and bustle of politics and economics and discipline. But the novel becomes a privileged place for the production of sexuality because it creates sex as a narrative secret that is simultaneously disclosed and buried by language, by literary form, and by novelistic themes.

The Gothic monster is an excellent example of the secret of sexuality that is both hidden and revealed within the same text. But the monster is also an example of the way that sexuality is constructed *as* identity in a way that ignores all other identifying traits (race, class, and gender to name a few). In *Frankenstein* the monster is pre-sexual, his sexuality, in other words, does not constitute his identity. But that is not to say that sexual aberration is missing from Shelley's definition of monstrosity: simply, sexuality is always a part of other identifying traits. For example, the monster's status as sexual outlaw and social pariah are mutually dependent. The endeavor of Frankenstein to first create life on his own and then to prevent his monster from mating suggests, if only by default, a homoerotic tension which underlies the incestuous bond. Franken-stein's voluntary exclusion from friends and family in pursuit of the secret of creating life also hints at the sexual nature of Victor's apparent withdrawal from all social intercourse. His creation of "a being like myself" hints at both masturbatory and homosexual desires which the scientist attempts to sanctify with the reproduction of another being. The suggestion that a homosexual bond in fact animates the plot adds an element of sexual perversity to the monster's already hybrid form.

In a feminist reading of Shelley's novel, Anne Mellor discusses the homoeroticism of the relationship between monster and author as part and parcel of patriarchal scientific ambition. Mellor argues that Victor is "engaged upon a rape of nature, a violent penetration and usurpation of the female's 'hiding places,' of the womb" and, she suggests, "in place of a heterosexual attachment to Elizabeth, Victor Frankenstein has substi-tuted a homosexual obsession with his creature."[14] Mellor's interpreta-tion of Victor Frankenstein's relation to his monster concludes that its homoerotics mask an implicit desire to create a race of men and, indeed, a world without women. Such a reading, however, runs the risk of sounding homophobic and misunderstands the relationship between homosexuality, textuality, and patriarchy.

In *Between Men* Eve Sedgwick attempts to define male homosocial desire in relation to homosexuality, homophobia, and the gender sys-tem. Her antihomophobic analysis leads her to deny "that patriarchal power is primarily or necessarily homosexual (as opposed to homoso-cial), or that male homosexual desire has a primary or necessary relation to misogyny."[15] Sedgwick's project — the disassociation of male homosociality from specifically male homosexual practices — allows us to distinguish between the activities of a persecuted sexual minority and the social relations between men upon which a system of dominance, patriarchy, rests. Since homophobia acts, then, as a control or check on all relations between men, the appearance of doubles and persecutory thematics in Gothic tells us more about fear than desire. As Sedgwick eloquently phrases it, ". . . paranoid Gothic is specifically not about homosexuals or the homosexual; instead heterosexuality is by definition its subject" (116). This claim corresponds very well to my claim that the novel is not about the making of a monster, its subject is the construction of humanness.

Sexual perversity and homosexual panic alone are not enough to characterize monstrosity. Sedgwick confirms that homophobia has a particular relation to the fear of femininity and that both play a part in class formations. Thus, the aristocracy, for example, a class in decline in the nineteenth century, may be feminized in relation to the "vigorous and productive values of the middle class" (93) and certain behaviors previously associated with aristocrats (as Sedgwick puts it, "effeminacy, connoisseurship, high religion" [93]) come to mark the homosexual. The sexually perverse can, in this way, be linked to a corrupt class (as it almost always was in early Gothic novels by Anne Radcliffe and Horace Walpole) and bad blood joins one to the other. But it is important to note the importance of race also within this topography of monstrosity; in the nineteenth century bad blood was becoming less and less a feature of old families and declining aristocrats and more an indicator of racial undesirability.

The connection between homosexuality and sociopolitical otherness can be made quite clear in terms of a belief in the inherent evil of certain groups of people. Hannah Arendt, in *The Origins of Totalitarianism,* makes the brilliant observation that crimes (the crime of being homosexual, the crime of being of the wrong race, i.e., Jewish) are turned into vices when a society is intent upon establishing a "world of fatalities."[16] In such a world Jews, for example, and homosexuals are bound by birth to their anomalous status and, as Arendt writes: "The seeming broad-mindedness that equates crime and vice, if allowed to establish its own code of law, will invariably prove more cruel and inhuman than laws, no matter how severe, which respect man's independent responsibility for his behavior" (82). The opposition between crime and vice is extremely important to an examination of Gothic monstrosity. Frankenstein's monster argues that his "vices are the children of a forced solitude" (147) but Victor thinks his monster, by virtue of his filthy form, was made to sin. Indeed, the equivocation between these two positions is unique to *Frankenstein* for, in the Gothic novel at the end of the nineteenth century, monsters are always born bad.

The homosexual subplot in *Frankenstein* props up an analogy between mixed blood and inherent perversity and suggests that while the "paranoid Gothic" is sustained on one level by a fear of sexuality between men, it also evinces a belief in the fixity of social relations and positions. Whatever disturbs these relations, this pattern, is "dirty" or "filthy" matter which must be excluded.[17] But in *Frankenstein* the complexity of the monster—it walks, it talks, it demands, it pursues, it rationalizes and shows emotion—confuses the politics of purity in which every dirty thing is marked and will pollute if not eliminated. The monster mixes humanity with physical deformity, a desire for community with an irreducible foreignness, great physical strength with femininity.

We recall that Frankenstein agrees to make the monster a mate because he has been somewhat moved by his creation's eloquent pleas for tolerance. When the monster confronts his maker amid the sublime scenery of the Alps, he moves his author to feel compassion and "a wish to console him" (147) but the sight of the monster still provokes horror: "when I saw the filthy mass that moved and talked, my heart sickened, and my feelings were altered to those of hatred and horror."[18] This sequence plays out what is, in the context of the novel, a by now familiar opposition between language and vision in which the visual registers horror while language confers humanity. Peter Brooks suggests that, in this episode, "we have an instance of what we might call, in the terms of Jacques Lacan, the imaginary versus the symbolic order." Brooks makes monstrosity thus an exclusion from signification and meaning; the monster may never accede into the symbolic, he is forever trapped by his hideous appearance in the imaginary.[19]

But monstrosity is not simply a matter of appearance, and perhaps the opposition between language and vision is more entangled than the model of "imaginary" and "symbolic" may imply. It is precisely in the realm of the symbolic, in the realm of language, of course, that monstrosity and humanity emerge as inseparable. The episode in which Frankenstein talks himself out of creating a female monster, for example, is remarkable for the way that it reconstructs the monster's monstrosity not simply as a visual production but as the place where the not-human is inscribed. The monster represents the inscription of the not-human through monstrosity, he is its textual form, his autobiography is the history of Gothic, as we shall see.

Sitting in his laboratory one evening during his efforts to make his monster a mate, Frankenstein ponders what he is doing. He begins to reason with himself about the morality of his new labors and he considers, "she might become ten thousand times more malignant than her mate," and "she might turn in disgust from him to the superior beauty of man," finally, "one of the first sympathies for which the daemon thirsted would be children, and a race of devils would be propagated upon the earth" (165). Here all compassion has been transformed into mistrustful fear. Frankenstein has not heard the monster's story at all and now he translates it into a demonic desire to populate the earth with a new race. Of course, Frankenstein is here engaged in what Freud would call "projection," the paranoid process by which "an internal perception is suppressed, and, instead, its content, after undergoing a certain degree of distortion, enters consciousness in the form of external perception."[20] Was it not Frankenstein himself who had hoped that his scientific breakthrough would make him the creator of a new species? "A new species would bless me as its creator and source; many happy and excellent natures would owe their being to me. No father could claim the gratitude of his child so completely as I should deserve theirs" (54). Projection literally transforms the monster into a screen, a place for the reinscription of monstrosity. While I will return to Freud's theory of "the mechanism of paranoia" in a later chapter, it is well to note here the mechanization of the human subject with relation to his conscious and unconscious behaviors.

Every time Frankenstein constructs his creation as monstrous, he renders invisible, immutable, and ineffable his own humanity. The self-evident nature of the "human" is constructed in Gothic as the destruction or inscription of the other. Visibility, I have been arguing, is the index of monstrosity in *Frankenstein* even as invisibility and ineffability imply humanity. Because of its readability, monstrosity allows us a peek at the construction of otherness out of the raw materials of racial undesirability, class definition, family ties, sexual perversity, and gender instability. The monster, therefore, by embodying what is not human, produces the human as a discursive effect. The human in *Frankenstein*, of course, is the Western European, bourgeois, male scientist. But monstrosity, I suggested early on, is inextricably bound to textuality, to the novelistic in particular, and so it is not surprising to discover that the history of Gothic monstrosity or embodied fear overlaps significantly with the history of the novel.

Pulp Fiction

The scene in which Victor decides to destroy the female monster is the most horrific, and indeed cinematic, episode in the novel. Unlike the first experiments which led Victor to discover the principle of life, the enterprise of building a female monster holds no romance for the scientist. When he first discovered "the cause of generation," Victor experienced "delight and rapture" (52) which only gave way to horror when he confronted the ugliness of his creation. Now, making a female, Victor finds every part of his work ugly and describes it as a "filthy process" (164). While, in the original experiments, Victor envisioned himself as a father to a "new species" and dreamed of achieving immortality, the idea of his monsters reproducing now seems like a curse that would cause "a race of devils to be propagated upon the earth" (165). As the thought occurs to him, the monster appears at the window and his "ghastly grin" resolves Victor to "destroy the creature on whose future existence he depended for happiness" (166).

In the aftermath of the destruction of the monster's mate, Victor sits frozen in his room and feels as if he is trapped in a nightmare. He hears steps approaching the door and wants to flee the inevitable meeting with the monster. Victor describes his inability to move: "I was overcome by the sensation of helplessness, so often felt in frightful dreams, when you in vain endeavor to fly from an impending danger" (167). After he had animated the male monster, Victor also suffered from nightmarish sensations and the scene of Elizabeth's murder on their wedding night by the monster takes on nightmarish proportions. After running in horror from the ugliness of his newly animated creation, Victor dreamt that he was embracing Elizabeth but his first kiss brought "the hue of death" to her features which then were transformed into those of his dead mother: "A shroud enveloped her form, and I saw the grave-worms crawling in the folds of the flannel" (58). In the hideous dismemberment of the female monster, Victor reenacts this scene from his nightmare; the bride-to-be (Elizabeth/the female monster) takes the nightmarish form of the dead mother. The meaning of Victor's dream is here clearly revealed to him —

Elizabeth merges with his mother in the nightmare not just as some oedipal fantasy but rather because monstrosity and maternity, in Victor's view, threaten always to join forces to reproduce a "race of devils."

The next day Victor returns to the laboratory and surveys the scene: "The remains of the half-finished creature, whom I had destroyed, lay scattered on the floor, and I almost felt as if I had mangled the living flesh of a human being" (170). Like the aftermath of a massacre in a modern splatter film, blood and flesh carpets the ground. Woman is reduced to a "half-finished creature" that man may take apart but not assemble. The making of a womb, apparently, challenges Victor with a scientific feat that he simply cannot and will not perform. He can build a man from the corpses of animals and humans but fashioning a woman demands that he construct and enervate a subject that is, in its future function at least, all body. The material horror of the female monster with her female genitals enrages and terrifies the scientist, he tears her limb from limb and scatters her flesh upon the ground.

The vision of Victor wrestling with the female flesh of the monster has the horrifying effect of a primal scene. The act of reproduction becomes here a bloody mess of dismemberment, a deconstruction of woman into her messiest and most slippery parts. As we noted in relation to the lumpen body of the male monster, the monster's body always is in a state of decomposition, it constantly threatens to unravel, to fail to hold together. In this scene deconstruction becomes a bloody act of violence, and a gendered violence at that.

The destruction of the female monster resembles, I noted, a primal scene. And yet, the mutilation of the female body is not satisfactorily explained by psychoanalysis. In a more productive discussion of female mutilation, Klaus Theweleit, in *Male Fantasies,* explains "two distinct processes at work in the acts of murder" carried out by fascist male soldiers on women. The first process equates assault with "a symbolic sexual act" and the second involves what he calls "the pleasurable perception of women in the condition of 'bloody masses.'"[21] Although Theweleit is discussing a particular historical phenomenon, his discussion of the soldiers' attitudes towards the mangled bodies of their female victims does have some bearing upon a discussion of Frankenstein's bloody murder of the female monster. Suggesting that the Freudian model of castration can only partly explain the impulse to murder defenseless women, Theweleit notes that once a woman has, within a certain psychological process, been stripped of all signs of identity, she can be "reduced to a pulp, a shapeless, bloody mass" (196). Far from being an erotic process, the dehumanization of woman, or indeed of any object — and this is something which Theweleit does not emphasize enough — the pulverizing of a body, even a monstrous body, is an act of radical indifference, an act which disregards the sexuality, indeed the physicality, of the flesh. Thus, while, as I have claimed, the violent destruction of the female monster may take on the proportions of a primal scene to the one who watches (the monster who views the flesh, in a way, as his flesh and blood), to the one who kills, the act of murder is merely a moral necessity, a compulsion to save the world from the contaminating potential of a "race of devils."

The murder of Elizabeth by the monster and the destruction of the female monster by Victor Frankenstein confirm that monstrosity is in the eye of the beholder. Both Victor and his monster have murdered, one out of moral compulsion, the other out of a frustrated desire for vengeance. The difference between the two acts seems slight and yet one, Victor's, is perhaps more terrifying and more revealing of the eventual direction of a politics of purity. The culmination of the process of dehumanization, whether it be directed towards monsters or men (and the difference between the two is merely a matter of perspective), produces a radical indifference towards the other as embodied subject. Victor views both the monster and his "half-finished" mate as "filthy mass," form without definition, desexualized matter, dirt. The only course of action which he feels can right the disturbed balance of the natural order is extermination. Victor pursues his "vampire" to the ends of the earth, finding only his own death in the arctic wasteland.

The bloody destruction of the female monster by Frankenstein has to be read alongside the sentimental narrative of family that centers upon Elizabeth and as a kind of metanarrative about Gothic itself. Elizabeth, indeed, pays in full for her fiancé's murderous desire, becoming a substitute for the female monster as the monster now directs his vengeance towards her. "I shall be with you on your wedding night," the monster warns his maker, as femininity and monstrosity are now merged into a single image of the desired woman. The domestic woman and the wild woman are both offered up as sacrificial victims to the masculinist narrative of discovery, invention, and competition.

The story of the female monster — a story within a story within a story — folds Gothic back upon itself. While certainly the image of one story folded into another suggests pregnancy, as Moers's essay on "female gothic" argues,[22] this is also a structure that firmly dissociates itself from the organic, the natural, and the reproductive. One story folded within another also signifies the machinic, the productive, the technological. The female monster—as basically the heart of the narrative beast, the central story in a spiraling narrative that spins into infinity—the female monster is the fleshy center that never speaks but always haunts the articulate narrative. She is at the opposite end of a structure that, as we recall, is framed by the invisible reader, Margaret Saville, and beyond that, of course, by the author herself, Mary Shelley.

When Frankenstein destroys the female mate of his monster, we witness an overdetermined moment that narrativizes the problem of definition embedded in the novel and the problem of population/popularity that makes the Gothic novel, as I am about to discuss, a feared symbol of mass culture. The female monster is mass like her mate, whom Frankenstein describes as a "sickening mass," and she becomes pulp as he grinds her flesh into oblivion. The fiction of pulp in this novel becomes a history of fiction and of its relation to gender and popular culture.

In a fascinating article on intersections of high and low culture within the Gothic, Bradford Mudge discusses the feminization of popular culture in the nineteenth century. Mudge makes provocative connections between the discourse on popular fiction and nineteenth-century discussions of prostitution. The coincidence of "the rise of the novel" with a growing population of female writers and readers has not always been acknowledged by conventional literary histories, Mudge suggests. To ignore gender when discussing a history of the novel, however, is to misunderstand the ways in which the growing tension between a high and a low culture at this time was inseparable from the growing participation of women in literary production and consumption.

Mudge cleverly links the intellectual threat that male critics felt from women's literary labor to the sexual threat posed by prostitutes to middle-class morality and he links both to a critique of capitalism: "Like eighteenth- and nineteenth-century prostitutes, who were both victims and perpetrators of entrepreneurial capitalism, women's novels enacted a transgression while upholding the very standard they transgressed: romance, domestic, and Gothic novels all competed successfully in a literary market that deplored market success as a criterion of value."[23] The popular novel, in such a discourse, is gendered as female, it is debased by the fact that it pleasures too many readers, and it is abused by the marketplace even as it prospers there. Mudge calls this the "feminization of popular culture."

There are two monsters, I have said, in *Frankenstein* and these two monsters, one male and one female, certainly symbolize different kinds of narratives. But the different narratives in *Frankenstein* do not simply break down into sentimental and Gothic, as at least one critic has suggested.[24] The female monster represents, in a way, the symbolic and generative power of monstrosity itself, and particularly of a monstrosity linked to femininity, female sexuality, and female powers of reproduction. For this reason we can read the female monster as a representative of exactly that threat that Mudge associates with popular culture in nineteenth-century England. While the male monster educates himself and argues eloquently with his maker, the female monster repels Frankenstein before he has even brought her to life. The male monster represents a sublimity which is missing from the female monster and while he becomes part of his author's identity, she threatens her maker with his own dissolution.

Terry Lovell, in *Consuming Fiction,* also challenges prevailing accounts of the rise of the novel within literary history. Lovell goes to work on Ian Watt's "seminal formulation of the thesis that the novel per se is essentially realist and bourgeois."[25] Lovell argues convincingly that we cannot identify the bourgeois novel only with realist conventions because it was clear that, between 1770 and 1820, bourgeois readers were also consuming vast quantities of Gothic Romance novels. Furthermore, she, like Mudge, points to the inadequacy of any history of the novel which does not account for the fact that women made up the majority of both writers and readers during the nineteenth century.

The rise of the novel, it is generally agreed, is linked to the development of capitalism. With the decline of literary patronage and the emergence of an anonymous literary marketplace, the novel was both commodified and produced according to the needs of capitalist ideology. However, by only identifying literary realism with capitalism, Lovell claims, theorists like Watt fail to account for the fact that "capitalism is Janus-faced." She writes:

> When the capitalist producer has his eye to his own management and work force, the qualities he likes to find and encourage are the classic bourgeois virtues — thrift, efficiency, hard work, frugality. But when he turns his attention to the purchaser of his commodities he may be happy to find a different creature, with money in wallet or purse and in a frame of mind to spend. . . . Bourgeois respectability and the contingencies of capitalist production create one kind of persona, capitalist consumption another. (31–32)

Capitalism, in other words, is dependent upon contradictions and there-fore plural in form; it demands an incoherent middle class with many different desires.

The Gothic novel, within Lovell's scheme, is a bourgeois form which caters to the consumer (rather than to the producer) and there-fore celebrates voluptuous excess and extravagance. We might take Lovell's argument one step further. As she points out, "consumer" was not exactly the right word for the book reader in the early nineteenth century because books were not exactly commodities (51). In order to cater to the consumer, then, the Gothic had to first produce the con-sumer and furthermore, produce the consumer as a productive identity. Since, later in the century, writers like Robert Louis Stevenson would write Gothic novels to earn some cash on the side and enable themselves to keep working on the less lucrative masterpieces, we must conclude that somewhere along the line the reader of fiction did become an active consumer. Gothic, I suggest, acted like an advertisement for the novel and *Frankenstein* was its most effective form. *Frankenstein* sells reading to a public and advertises interpretation by presenting the text as a monster that must be identified, decoded, captured, and consumed.

Frankenstein does precisely teach readers to read and encourages readers to think of themselves as readers and to take pleasure in the activity. Because the text is presented to the reader as a puzzle and be-cause, as Lovell points out, "the narrative lacks . . . any character who can stand in for the imputed reader" (59), reading becomes an activity that generates its own pleasures, the pleasures of the text. The novel, then, as a commodity, as a form of knowledge, can be called Gothic when and where it locates its own function as a monstrous productivity and con-nects that function to a host of fears associated with popularity, popula-tion, consumerism, mass culture, femininity, the foreign, class wars, and sexual perversion.

The reduction of the female monster to pulp gives us a very literal metaphor for the threat of female monstrosity as opposed to the threat figured by male monstrosity. The pulp that Frankenstein scatters about his laboratory floor *is* the female monster, is female monstrosity. It is both a fleshy sexuality that Frankenstein originally fled from by leaving his home, his mother, and his bride to be and also formless flesh that refuses to become human. The power of the male monster is that it does precisely become human and so it makes humanity intrinsic to a particu-lar kind of monstrosity and vice versa. The female monster cannot be human because it is always only an object, a thing, "unfinished."

If we extend this analysis of the female monster's metaphoric value, it is possible to argue for the female monster as pulp fiction within the allegory of literary production that Shelley has given us. We are entitled to read the novel as allegory because her introduction makes the connection for the reader between book and monster, maker and author. The book that the female monster represents is not the book that we read, it is the popular narrative that escapes into popular consciousness as the myth of Frankenstein. It is formless and endlessly repeatable.

Gothic Realism

Looking ahead to twentieth-century Gothic horror, a narrative that resides almost exclusively in popular cinema, one finds that the female monster lives on as the victim of male violence who is endlessly constructed and destroyed, violated and remade. For example, the female monster may be traced to the discarded flesh of Buffalo Bill's victims in *The Silence of the Lambs* (1991); since this murderer is only interested in female skins, he dumps the flesh within into his bathtub like garbage. Or she is the transvested mother in Hitchcock's *Psycho;* with the mother long dead, Anthony Perkins becomes his mother but keeps her remains in a basement. She is the dead grandmother in *The Texas Chainsaw Massacre 2* who sits above ground with her chain saws across her chest keeping watch over the family fortunes. The female monster is a pile of "remains," the leftover material, the excess of the narrative, the excess that renders the narrative Gothic. Interestingly enough, in the conventional Gothic novels of the 1890s, the male monster dominates as an almost heroic figure, the female monster is present on the margins but she does not signify in her own body the power of horror, she signifies its limits, its boundaries.

To trace the female monster in the time that intervenes between *Frankenstein* and the modern horror film, we have to search the basements and the attics of the nineteenth-century realist novel. She is Bertha Mason in *Jane Eyre,* the ghost of Cathy in *Wuthering Heights,* she is often the prostitute or lower-class servant. And in the novels of Charles Dickens, the female monster inhabits the heart of the city as Nancy, as the woman who lures men to evil ends. Although the Gothic itself after Shelley seems to disappear for eighty years as a distinct genre, it lives on throughout the nineteenth century as the dark heart of a realism that is always, to some degree, Gothic.

3

Gothic Surface, Gothic Depth: The Subject
of Secrecy in Stevenson and Wilde

*[M]an is not truly one but two, I say two because the state of my own knowledge
does not pass beyond that point. Others will follow, others will outstrip me on the
same lines; and I hazard the guess that man will be ultimately known for a mere
polity of multifarious, incongruous, and independent denizens.* — THE STRANGE
CASE OF DR. JEKYLL AND MR. HYDE

*Insincerity . . . is merely a method by which we can multiply our personalities.
Such . . . was Dorian Gray's opinion. He used to wonder at the shallow psychology
of those who conceived the Ego in man as a thing simple, permanent, reliable,
and of one essence. To him man was a being with myriad lives and myriad sensations, a complex, multiform creature . . .* — THE PICTURE OF DORIAN GRAY

Gothic Humanism

The post-Frankenstein monster emerges at the turn of the century
as a creature marked by an essential duality and a potential multiplicity.
While we remarked that the monster in *Frankenstein* is always part of his
maker, always also constructing his author, the dialectic between monster and maker is resolved in both Robert Louis Stevenson's *Dr. Jekyll
and Mr. Hyde* (1886) and Oscar Wilde's *The Picture of Dorian Gray*
(1891) as a conflict staged in a single body. If the monster's monstrosity
in *Frankenstein* depended upon the fragility of his maker's humanity, the
hideous nature of Mr. Hyde can only be known through the failed respectability of Dr. Jekyll, and the decrepitude of Dorian's portrait is only
significant when juxtaposed to his own youthful beauty.

In order to understand why the monster returns as two monsters, it
is helpful and necessary to compare Robert Louis Stevenson's shilling
shocker to its twin tale, Wilde's *The Picture of Dorian Gray*. The two

novels play out the drama of Dr. Jekyll and Mr. Hyde by presenting the same history but in very different forms — one is, as Stevenson put it, a "Gothic gnome,"[1] stunted, cramped, ugly and designed to shock not soothe; the other is beautiful, artistic, born of aesthetics. In each book Gothic effect depends upon the production of a monstrous double and in each the plot resolves itself into a tidy (if unconvincing) moral resolution. Furthermore, both novels were dubbed "poisonous" by reviewers and were reviled for both their forms and their subject matter.

"Man is not truly one but truly two. . . ." says Dr. Jekyll as he pursues his scientific experimentation. *Dr. Jekyll and Mr. Hyde* uses multiple narrators to tell the story of a man doomed by the chemical reproduction of his double. Dr. Jekyll, we learn, is a man tormented by a sense of the essential duplicity of his being and, indeed, by a sense of "the thorough and primitive duality of man."[2] Jekyll embarks upon what he conceives of as a moral and scientific project, the dissociation of the "polar twins" of the self. Experimenting with various chemical compounds, Jekyll discovers a potion which, when he imbibes it, transforms his body into that of his other self. The other self, Mr. Hyde, enacts Jekyll's undignified desires and haunts the streets of London, a small and dark, indescribably ugly character. Hyde's menacing aspect and his violent ways lead him to murder and Jekyll vows never to drink the transformative potion again. The metamorphosis, however, has become spontaneous and Jekyll feels his respectable side succumbing to the evil of his double. The story unfolds through the narratives of Jekyll's lawyer, John Gabriel Utterson; his friend and colleague, Dr. Lanyon; and finally the last testament of Jekyll himself. The various narratives combine to create a mystery, the mystery surrounding Hyde — who is he, where did he come from, why is he so evil, what is his connection to the good Dr. Jekyll — which can only be solved after Jekyll's death when Utterson reads the papers he leaves behind.

In Oscar Wilde's *The Picture of Dorian Gray,* a young man sells his soul to be eternally youthful while a portrait of him grows old in his place. Under the tutelage of Lord Henry Wotton, a cynic and a man of leisure, Dorian learns to take immense pleasure in a superficial life. While his painting takes on the appearance of depth, Dorian remains a perfect surface, a canvas stretched across a soul. Lord Henry appears as a kind of Frankenstein figure in this narrative and he sees Dorian as a live experiment in "natural science": "To a large extent the lad was his own creation. He had made him premature. That was something."[3] But Dorian is also Basil Hallward's creation since Basil paints his portrait and thus divides him against himself. When he saw the portrait for the first time, Dorian "drew back and his cheeks flushed for a moment with pleasure. A look of joy came into his eyes, as if he had recognized himself for the first time" (24). Dorian's desire to be the self he sees in the picture dooms him.

By reading Stevenson's Gothic gnome alongside Wilde's "poisonous book," I hope to read one as an inversion of the other and both as Gothic narratives of a self marked, not by its fear of the other, but by a paranoid terror of involution or the unraveling of a multiformed ego. But this is not a psychological study, not a psychoanalysis of these two dual egos; this is a history of subject formation within the Gothic narrative which examines why and how these narratives seem to insist upon psychological interpretations and why and how such psychological readings already assume the self that is in fact in the process of being constructed within the horror story. In other words, *Dr. Jekyll and Mr. Hyde* creates a self within the self, it constructs a depth to subjectivity, but we are prone to read it as a description of the conflict between man's inner and outer being. *The Picture of Dorian Gray,* however, works backwards; it critiques the notion that subjectivity is a deep structure and it demands that we stay "shallow," that we remain at the surface, that we take surface as truth, that we understand truth as always superficial, and that we cultivate instead an understanding of subjectivity based upon the lie.

Critics have a tendency to read *Dr. Jekyll and Mr. Hyde* in particular as a morality tale about Victorian hypocrisy. Martin Tropp, for example, in *Images of Fear,* compares the myth of Jack the Ripper and the fiction told by Stevenson in *Dr. Jekyll and Mr. Hyde* in terms of the violence produced by a contradiction between outward appearance and inner reality: "*Dr. Jekyll and Mr. Hyde* became a blueprint for speculation about the murders because both events—fictional and factual—conveyed, graphically and undeniably, a sense of the precariousness of a culture caught between outward respectability and secret violence."[4] Hypocrisy, however, the tension between "outward respectability" and "secret violence," already assumes too much about the shared monstrosity of a Dr. Jekyll and Jack the Ripper. It assumes that the humanity of the subject, for example, is founded upon the three-dimensional form of subjecthood. It assumes that a surface of respectability is antithetical to a hidden violence. But perhaps it is only the modern reader who understands "respectable" to mean "nonviolent"; Stevenson's story makes the violent, the criminal, and the destructive continuous with the respectable surface.

Tropp, indeed, in an effort to be historical, has precisely transcended history by making historical categories like "respectability" a cause rather than an effect of cultural narratives about Gothic selves. Tropp continues: "Stevenson's private nightmare and Whitechapel's public reality were parallel events and together foreshadowed the way the modern world has come to view human possibility. Random, purposeless violence is the ultimate horror of the city in the twentieth century, a horror made possible by urban anonymity and the loss of community" (130). The idea of a foreshadowing and a consequent production of a new horror, of course, constructs a mythical time "before" when there was a community (that is now lost) and a more optimistic view of "human possibility." I propose that we read one Gothic narrative, *Dr. Jekyll and Mr. Hyde,* inside another, *The Picture of Dorian Gray,* and allow the one to unravel the other precisely so that we may avoid a transhistorical and humanist reading of Gothic. Certainly fictional horror and factual horror are in some kind of dialogue but they are not merely symptoms of the decay and essential monstrosity of humanness. Rather, they are narratives that produce ideological and interpretive strategies for readers to recognize the human and distinguish between human and monster.

Gothic Gnomes

Stevenson viewed *Dr. Jekyll and Mr. Hyde* as a "shilling shocker" or "a fine bogey tale"[5] written very quickly to earn money. In an essay on the mass readership of the Victorian period, Patrick Brantlinger and Richard Boyle take Stevenson's comments to refer to the double bind of the artist torn between writing literary masterpieces and making money. Stevenson, they suggest, struggles with the notion that if his work is widely read then it must be deformed or it must resemble the sensationalist "yellow press" of the day. They write: "Stevenson as popular author shares in the criminal 'popularity' or populace-like nature of Hyde. 'There must be something wrong with me.' The statement is, in a sense, the formula of *Dr. Jekyll and Mr. Hyde* itself. There is 'something wrong' in the story — that is Hyde — and this accounts for its popularity" (274). Bratlinger and Boyle provide a provocative analysis of Stevenson's conception of his own popularity and they dissect the opposition of popularity and the literary and the juxtaposition of Gothic and deformity implicit in Stevenson's disdain of his "Gothic gnome." What exactly *is* wrong with Mr. Hyde is not so easily explained, however, since he seems to be wrong in a multitude of ways. Like Frankenstein's monster, Mr. Hyde is visually repellent but unlike Frankenstein's monster, his repulsive nature extends beyond his exterior. Hyde is born bad and he is bad through and through; he also represents the evil core of his author, Mr. Jekyll.

Both Stevenson's book and Hyde are Gothic gnomes in that Hyde is "dwarfish" (18) and "ape-like" (27) and has a "haunting sense of unexpressed deformity" (32); and the novel is very short, a kind of stunted work which, despite the obvious moral overtones, concerns itself with the dark recesses of the city and the self. The novel's very popularity announces it as nonliterary within a Victorian context and its appeal for a mass audience suggests that it must fail to satisfy the high cultural expectations that critics like Matthew Arnold espoused.[6]

Stevenson's identification of his "shilling shocker" with the monstrous Hyde is reminiscent of an earlier connection made by Mary Shelley between book and monster when she dubbed *Frankenstein* "my hideous progeny." We might say, in fact, that the merger of book and monster is a typical Gothic strategy but it is also an identification that is repeated in many histories of the novel which make the Gothic a kind of degenerate cousin to the realist novel.[7] Gothic novels, indeed, play monster to the three-volume masterpiece that represented art or culture in the nineteenth century.[8] Like other Gothic novels, *Dr. Jekyll and Mr. Hyde* is not a "masterpiece" but a "monsterpiece" and, ironically, it tells the story of a monster hiding in the master.

Like *Dr. Jekyll and Mr. Hyde* and like *Frankenstein,* a mainstay of *The Picture of Dorian Gray* is the connection that Wilde makes between art and monstrosity. The obvious metaphor of monstrous textuality in the novel is the picture of Dorian Gray painted by Basil Hallward who is in love with him. Dorian wishes one day that "the face on the canvas bear the burden of his passions and his sins," that it, instead of him, should grow old. His wish is granted and the portrait becomes a record of his life, his desires, his corruption while he retains the bloom of youth and purity. But there is also another metaphor for corrupt artistic production in this novel — the "poisonous book" that Lord Henry Wotton sends to Dorian, now his protégé.

Even though Wilde made it clear that his story is a morality play about the intersections of life and art, the public reception of *The Picture of Dorian Gray* still turned the novel into a monster. *The Picture of Dorian Gray* was immediately slandered by the press as "poisonous," as filled with "odors of moral and spiritual putrefaction," as obsessed with "disgusting sins and abominable crimes."[9] Wilde responded to such criticism by claiming that, far from being an immoral tale, his book was in fact too moral. He writes in a letter to the editor of *The Daily Chronicle*: "My story is an essay on decorative art. It reacts against the crude brutality of plain realism. It is poisonous if you like, but you cannot deny that it is also perfect. . . ."[10] The "poisonous book" that infects Dorian is supposedly Huysman's *Against Nature* and it is described in the text as a "yellow book" and as "the strangest novel he had ever read. . . . It was a novel without a plot" (125). The "yellow" novel becomes an obvious metaphor for Wilde's novel itself but it also becomes an uncanny double for the kind of monstrosity that Gray represents. Like the book, Dorian is "perfect," he is all form and no content. Dorian is in some sense plotless because his life is not written upon his body but upon his portrait. He is beautiful but all surface and without depth.

The allegory of artistic production that both *The Picture of Dorian Gray* and *Dr. Jekyll and Mr. Hyde* tell makes the process of narration itself Gothic. While the "poisonous book" in *The Picture of Dorian Gray* is offensive because it has no plot, the picture of Dorian is hideous because it has too much plot and these two sources of disgust are both made more hideous by the fact of Dorian's own perfect beauty. Similarly, the relationship between Dr. Jekyll and Mr. Hyde is that of a terrible dependency between author and text (and Jekyll is depicted as a junky addicted to his chemical production). Hyde is born of Jekyll and yet, Jekyll's narrative, the authentic, realist, and conventional tale of a good man's undoing, is organized by and mandated by Hyde's tale. In the process of telling, of course, the Gothic and the realist stories become completely entangled and instead of resolving themselves into two different lines of logic, they rise and fall together. Indeed, the narrative trajectories in both novels lead inexorably towards the blending of one identity into the other. Jekyll comments: "All things therefore seemed to point to this; that I was slowly losing hold of my original and better self, and slowly becoming incorporated with my second and worse" (90).

The profound entanglement of identities and genres in both of the novels I am discussing here suggests that textual identities mesh with physical identities and bodies are bound up in souls and perversions are inextricably wedded to respectability and evil or immoral activity is continuous with what we call human. The task of each of these novels, however, is to unwind the messy skein of identities and separate out the good from the ugly, the bad from the pure, the perverted from the kind, the sexual from the spiritual, the beautiful from the unhealthy. But as much as the texts seem to manipulate and stretch their monsters, pulling them further and further from the jeopardy of "human" identity, the more the tendency is towards chaos. Monsters, texts, sexualities, and identities seem, like Hyde, to retract automatically to the "slime of the pit" (100) and, like Jekyll, they are always in danger of transformation. For the brief moments that monster does stand apart from human we catch a glimpse of the construction of identities and we witness the ways in which Gothic deploys monstrosity to condense negative meaning into bodies with highly specific sexual, racial, and class codings. This chapter attempts to read the ghostly apparitions of homosexual, Jew, and woman when and where they enter and leave the site of monstrosity.

Dress and Disguise

The monster is always a master of disguise and his impermanence and fleeting sense of reality precisely marks him as monstrous. In *Dr. Jekyll and Mr. Hyde,* Stevenson makes disguise a structural principle as well as a thematic. He blurs completely the generic specificity that was supposed to separate the literature of vulgarity from the literature of "sweetness and light" and indeed, he disguises one as the other (the Gothic tale is disguised as a moral fable; the moral fable is disguised as a monster story) but it becomes impossible to decide what or who is dressed as what or whom. This story, like *The Picture of Dorian Gray,* is finally a costume drama.

Some contemporary reviews of Stevenson's *Dr. Jekyll and Mr. Hyde* call attention to the peculiarity of this novel's form and content and to the sense that, like Jekyll/Hyde, the novel itself is somehow in disguise. Henry James, for example, uses very specifically sartorial metaphors to describe Stevenson's writing: "There are writers who present themselves before the critic with just the right amount of drapery that is necessary for decency; but Mr Stevenson is not one of those—he makes his appearance in an amplitude of costume. His costume is part of his character . . . it never occurs to us to ask how he would look without it. Before all things he is a writer with style."[11] James here makes literary style into a "costume" that both cloaks the writer and his subject but that also becomes integral to the writer's identity. Elsewhere Stevenson himself refers to literary form as "so much plastic material."[12] But note that, in terms of Gothic writing, literary language is described in terms of its "amplitude," its excess. Gothic seems to denote the clothed word as opposed to the near nakedness of supposed realist writing which hesitates to call attention to its costume.

We might almost say that the grotesque effect of Gothic is achieved through a kind of transvestism, a dressing up that reveals itself as costume. Gothic is a cross-dressing, drag, a performance of textuality, an infinite readability and, indeed, these are themes that are readily accessible within Gothic fiction itself where the tropes of doubling and disguise tend to dominate the narrative. If we apply this Jamesian metaphor of the cross-dressed word to *Dr. Jekyll and Mr. Hyde,* we have to situate Jekyll as a man who fits comfortably into his own clothes and is a metaphor for the realist writing that presents itself "with just the right amount of drapery that is necessary for decency." Hyde, on the other hand, appears at one point in the novel dressed in Jekyll's clothes and they seem to drown him because they are too big for him. Hyde represents the outrageously dressed up Gothic horror, a monster in lawyer's clothes. But he is also the costume that Jekyll assumes at times. Jekyll remarks: "I had but to drink the cup, to doff at once the body of the noted professor and to assume, like a thick cloak, that of Edward Hyde" (85). He also refers to Hyde as a form that he "wears" (90).

Writing is characterized very specifically as disguise in *Dr. Jekyll and Mr. Hyde.* Handwriting, at several points in the narrative, is held up as a witness to identity. In one scene Utterson's head clerk, "a great student and critic of handwriting" (38), is given an opportunity to compare Dr. Jekyll's handwriting with that of his "minion," Mr. Hyde. Guest comes quickly to the conclusion that "there's a rather singular resemblance; the two hands are in many points identical: only differently sloped" (39). Here autographs and signatures become the inscriptions of a dual identity and one is assumed to be a forgery of the other. But of course, both identities and neither of them are forged; each one depends upon the hidden presence of the other and each must perform and inscribe the doubleness and instability of the identity they share. Moving back and forth between these two tales, one of Dr. Jekyll and one of Mr. Hyde, the text alternates between the two differently sloped handwritings as one tale constantly disguises or writes over the other. Jekyll's tragic tale of decline is underwritten by Hyde's sensational story of murder and mayhem. Hyde's struggle to liberate himself from the repressive force of the doctor is overcome by Jekyll's attempt to return to the cozy nest of professional camaraderie represented by his friends Utterson and Lanyon. The realist story of a good doctor striving for knowledge is shot through with the Gothic tale of sexual outrage and physical violence. Never one without the other.

In case the cross-dressing performance that Gothic represents (Gothic as a perverse costume that the realist story is dressed up in) seems obscure, let us return to James's analysis of Stevenson's style. Having drawn the analogy between style and costume, he goes one step further: "Mr. Stevenson delights in a style, and his has nothing accidental or diffident; it is eminently conscious of its responsibilities and meets them with a kind of gallantry — as if language were a pretty woman, and a person who proposes to handle it had of necessity be something of a Don Juan" (141). The significant aspect of this passage, of course, lies in James's characterization of language as a "pretty woman," as feminine, as ornamentation that treads that thin line between pretty and garish. An "amplitude of costume" in such an analogy suggests a dangerous proximity both to prostitution (dressed to sell perhaps, keeping in mind that Stevenson wrote *Dr. Jekyll and Mr. Hyde* hoping to make some money from its sales) but also to a grotesque transvestism. James continues his analysis of the writer as a Don Juan in relation to the seductive allure of "pretty" literary language:

> The bravery of gesture is a noticeable part of his nature, it is rather odd that at the same time a striking feature of that nature should be an absence of care for things feminine. His books are for the most part books without women, and it is not women who fall most in love with them. But Mr. Stevenson does not need, as we might say, a petticoat to inflame him: a happy collocation of words will serve the purpose. (141)

Again, this is a curiously inflected passage in which James wants to claim the romantic proclivities of a Don Juan for Stevenson while noting that women seem to neither interest nor be interested in him. What serves as his love object in this passage is language itself, and a language moreover which is characterized by femininity and which can therefore allow the author to "achieve his best effects without the aid of the ladies."

I will claim here that Gothic, the "amplitude of costume" and the feminine guise which is worn by an author, plays homosexual to the healthy and appropriately garbed heterosexuality of realism. Gothic is the debased and degenerate cousin who calls too much attention to himself by an outrageous and almost campy performance of all of the tricks of the literary trade. Gender and genre here, and genre and sexuality, slide into each other as plasticity of form comes to define gender, genre, and sexual identity. But, as I will show in my discussion of the cross-dressing Gothic-homo performances of Jekyll, Hyde, and Dorian Gray, Gothic reveals the ideological stakes of a bourgeois realism — namely, there is no one generic form that resembles "life" and another debased form that deviates from the natural order of things. There are only less or more fantastic costumes, less or more Gothic interpretations of reality. As Arthur Symons said of Stevenson, "He was never really himself except when he was in some fantastic disguise."[13] The fantastic disguises in *Dr. Jekyll and Mr. Hyde* and *The Picture of Dorian Gray* are precisely what make each character "really himself."

Disguise in *The Picture of Dorian Gray* is a little more complicated but it just as obviously becomes a trope for homoerotic desire. We need to read dress and disguise in this novel against the backdrop of decadence. Oscar Wilde, of course, is considered to be one of the main representatives of the decadent movement in England and the protagonists of *The Picture of Dorian Gray* embody the kinds of attitudes and demeanors that were popularly associated with decadence and dandyism. Some scholars, like Regenia Gagnier, link dandyism to "high Society" and the aristocracy. But Richard Dellamora, in *Masculine Desire,* claims that the dandy has been misidentified or "misplaced": "Although some aristocrats were dandies, the 'dandy' as a popular phenomenon is middle-class. . . . Dandyism was associated with middle-class uppityism . . . dandyism also reflects a loss of balance between the dual imperatives of leisure and work incumbent upon Victorian gentlemen. The dandy is too relaxed, too visible, consumes to excess while producing little or nothing."[14] The dandy is also, as Dellamora makes clear, too feminine. He unites, then, the threat of idleness and a delinquent femininity in a male form that is marked by its desire to be noticed.

The dandy, of course, is a Gothic monster in the context of Oscar Wilde's narrative about the beautiful Dorian Gray. Like the monstrosity of Frankenstein's creature or of Hyde, the horror exerted by the dandy is multipurpose and primarily visual. He represents too much and too little, excess and paucity; the dandy represents the parasitical aristocrat and the upwardly mobile bourgeois. He obviously also represents the homosexual male.[15] Wilde characterizes Dorian's dandyism in terms of his fashion sense: "Fashion, by which what is really fantastic becomes for a moment universal, and dandyism, which in its own way, is an attempt to assert the absolute modernity of beauty, had, of course, their fascination for him" (129). His "fashion" sense, his charm, his foppery make Dorian a monster because they allow him to seduce men and women alike with his appearance of perfect purity. Vampirelike, Dorian lives upon the desire he consumes from his lovers and he revels in the contrast between his own beauty and "the evil and aging face on the canvas" (128). As his body becomes more and more a fashion plate, a place to hang costumes, so the canvas devolves more and more into sin and corruption.

Dorian's affair with Sibyl Vane reveals the real stakes that Wilde's narrative has in costume and disguise. Early on in the story, Dorian falls in love with a young actress. When he first sees her, Sibyl is playing Juliet, another time she is Rosalind "wandering through the forest of Arden, disguised as a pretty boy in hose and doublet and dainty cap" (51). Dorian desires the girl obviously for her performances, and particularly for her transvestite performances, and he asks Lord Henry ironically, "Harry! why didn't you tell me that the only thing worth loving is an actress?" (51). Sibyl's appeal for Dorian lies completely in her ability to be all the "great heroines of the world in one" and never simply Sibyl Vane. She is even able to be some of the "pretty boys" of the world. But when she reveals herself to be just plain Sibyl Vane, Dorian feels that she has "killed my love" (86). "You," she says, "taught me what reality really is. Tonight, for the first time, I saw through the hollowness, the sham, the silliness of the empty pageant in which I had always played" (86). And it is precisely when the boundaries between the spheres of art and life are too clearly drawn that desire, for Dorian, disappears.

For Dorian, and one presumes for Wilde, the surface is all that identity consists of. As Wilde quips in his preface: "Those who go beneath the surface do so at their own peril." Going beneath the surface is certainly perilous in the context of the novel where Sibyl Vane and Basil both die because they attempt to break through superficialities and arrive at something "real." Sibyl, of course, thinks that theater masks life and Basil believes that art idealizes life. Each one attempts to move decisively from one realm of meaning to the other, from illusion to reality, but each discovers that the penalty for making too neat a distinction between art and life is death. When he learns of Sibyl's death, Dorian says: "How extraordinarily dramatic life is! If I had read all this in a book, Harry, I think I would have wept over it. Somehow now that it has actually happened, and to me, it seems far too wonderful for tears" (98). Dorian, like Harry, never mistakes life for reality; he recognizes that life is more dramatic than theater and he is rewarded with longevity.

In both *The Picture of Dorian Gray* and *Dr. Jekyll and Mr. Hyde,* disguise becomes equivalent to self in a way that confuses the model of subjectivity that each author maps. While at first the model of a monster hiding behind a respectable or aesthetically pleasing front seems to produce a deep, structured subjectivity, in each the hidden self subverts the notion of an authentic self and makes subjectivity a surface effect. The important difference between disguise or illusion in *The Picture of Dorian Gray* and *Dr. Jekyll and Mr. Hyde* lies perhaps in their conceptions of what lies beneath the costume. In *Dr. Jekyll and Mr. Hyde,* it is obvious that Hyde is precisely the base costume, the foundation, for Jekyll. When Jekyll chemically produces Hyde, he peels back a layer of respectability and exposes what lay hidden (I'll return to the pun on "hide" later). But Dorian's relation to his portrait is a variation upon a surface and depth model; the portrait is all surface but it gives the illusion of depth once it has begun to record the rotting of Dorian's soul. Furthermore, as Jeff Nunokawa points out, in *The Picture of Dorian Gray,* "the expression of homosexual desire cancels, rather than clarifies, the definition of the character through whom it is conducted" (313). The friction of surfaces, in other words, in this text is as likely to erase self as it is to construct another one. Each novel produces a form of Gothic subjectivity, that is to say, each text presents the ego as "multi-formed," as either a series of shifting surfaces or a volume of buried depths. The relation between surface and depth in Wilde's novel is produced as a sexual relation.

Secrets, Sex, and Surfaces

The profound ugliness of Mr. Hyde is perhaps matched only by the exquisite and perfect beauty of Dorian Gray, a youth who "was certainly wonderfully handsome, with his finely-curved scarlet lips, his frank blue eyes, his crisp gold hair" (15). But both Hyde and Gray represent a similar threat, the sexual menace of perverse desire and the epistemological menace of unstable identities. Extreme beauty and extreme ugliness are thus both linked to sexual perversity and specifically to homosexual proclivities but they are also framed as disguises for unspeakable crimes. In terms of Mr. Hyde, perversity has dragged his physical form down to its most base constituents and in Dorian Gray homosexuality announces itself as pure beauty unsullied by moral or ethical consideration.

In *The Picture of Dorian Gray*, and particularly in the subplot of the romance between Dorian and Sibyl Vane, Wilde associates homosexuality with illusion and heterosexuality with reality. So, for example, Dorian rejects Sibyl when he discovers his own preference for illusion and artifice over reality. She, however, would abandon her acting career for the love of a man. Basil, too, loved illusion and the secret of his painting of Dorian is that "I am afraid I have shown in it the secret of my soul" (4). He guards his soul and his painting, refusing to show either in public, and he comments, "I have grown to love secrecy. It seems to be the one thing that can make modern life mysterious or marvelous" (4). Lord Henry obviously cares nothing for reality. He makes everything into an act. "Being natural," he quips, "is simply a pose" (5).

Eve Sedgwick has made homosexuality an integral feature of Gothic horror. She calls attention to the paranoid Gothic as a genre fraught with tension between "normal" relations between men and perverse sexual relations between men. In Gothic, slippage occurs between these two already unstable categories and the monster, or the agent of fear, becomes easily recognizable as queer: "The Gothic novel crystallized for English audiences the terms of a dialectic between male homosexuality and homophobia, in which homophobia appeared thematically in paranoid plots."[16] Sedgwick points out that many of the early Gothic Romance authors were linked in one way or another to some homosexual scandal (Lewis was openly homosexual, Beckford was driven out of England for homosexual philandering, Walpole was linked to homosexual attachments). Homosexuality, still according to Sedgwick, becomes equivalent to the unspeakable in Gothic Romance and, we might add, by the end of the century, secret and unlawful desires are euphemisms for homosexuality. The secret and sexuality are forever linked, of course, by the 1890s legislations against homosexual activity and, as we will see, by the 1890s medicalization of sexuality.

Homoerotic bonds between men, indeed, animate both novels and propel them towards the discovery of secret selves. Jekyll keeps a secret self locked away, a self that is defiled because it has "forbidden desires." Male sexuality in both stories represents mirrored and narcissistic effect which, as we see also in *The Picture of Dorian Gray,* is both homoerotic and paranoid—paranoid because of the panic unleashed by the recognition of desire between men. Both novels are populated mostly by men who meet secretly, dine together, spend hours together. The opening scene of *Dr. Jekyll and Mr. Hyde* depicts Enfield and Utterson on one of their Sunday walks: "[T]he two men put the greatest store by these excursions, counted them the chief jewel of each week, and not only set aside occasions of pleasure, but even resisted the calls of business that they might enjoy them uninterrupted" (2). Homosexuality haunts both *Dr. Jekyll and Mr. Hyde* and *The Picture of Dorian Gray.* If Jekyll and Hyde are cross-dressing monsters slipping in and out of each other's clothes, Dorian Gray is the monster who never changes. His distilled beauty is the hallmark of his perversity, however, and the secret to his beauty becomes his sexual secret. The outrage that Gothic novels produce has everything to do with telling secrets. Again, *The Picture of Dorian Gray* thematizes this preoccupation—it is about secrets but it hesitates to actually tell anything. We do not learn, for example, the exact nature of Dorian's various crimes or the reasons for his friend Chambers's death or Henry Wotton's sister's death; we only know that Wilde has caused them. The hidden self of Dorian Gray is indeed a sexual self, a decadent self, a self too much preoccupied with art, representation, and beauty rather than life, experience, the common lot.

Furthermore, a set of behaviors that earlier in the century had characterized the corruption of the aristocracy (Mr. Fairlie in Wilkie Collins's *The Woman in White,* for example)—effeminacy, sensuality, love of art, uselessness, idle leisured existence—now came to stereotype homosexual behavior. While aristocrats were denigrated as parasites upon the middle-class capitalists—they produced nothing and did nothing "useful"—homosexuals were seen as nonproductive, fruitless, given over to the reproduction of art not life. The queer dandyism that Wilde exemplified, furthermore, emphasized the artificial over the real, art over life, and connected aestheticism to self-advertisement and an essential male femininity.[17]

Dorian Gray is singled out first by Basil Hallward and then by Lord Henry Wotton as the perfect object for artistic and aesthetic contemplation. Basil's desire for Dorian is immediately annexed to secrecy. He attempts, in the novel's opening scene, to keep Dorian Gray's name from Henry. In order for something to be desired in this novel, it must also be forbidden and silenced. Basil immediately connects the painting of Dorian Gray to "the secret of my own soul" and fears that he must not show it because he will reveal his soul. It is not until much later that he tells Dorian his "secret": "But I know that as I worked at it, every flake and film of colour seemed to me to reveal my secret. I grew afraid that others would know of my idolatry. I felt, Dorian, that I had told too much, that I had put too much of myself into it" (114). Basil's secret is his love for Dorian as art object, his love for beauty, and his love for male beauty in particular. While Basil's secret, then, is his desire for Dorian, Dorian's secret is his own portrait. Desire, in this narrative, one might say, is the secret that art tells and that the subject conceals.

Secrecy, in *Dr. Jekyll and Mr. Hyde,* is irrevocably annexed to the persona of Mr. Hyde. Hyde's name and his desire to roam the streets at night mark him as one who must always move under cover. Jekyll, also, is perceived as under cover or masked, however, when his servants spot Hyde in Jekyll's clothes. Poole, Dr. Jekyll's manservant, calls upon Utterson and asks him to come and intervene between Jekyll and his mysterious laboratory work. Poole tells Utterson that he thinks someone other than Jekyll resides in the laboratory and he tells of his fright upon seeing this person emerge. But, asks Utterson, how do you know it was not Jekyll? Poole replies: "Sir, if that was my master, why had he a mask upon his face? If that was my master, why did he cry out like a rat, and run from me? I have served him long enough. . . . My master . . . is a tall, fine build of a man, and this was more of a dwarf" (56). Later Poole adds, "There was something queer about that gentleman . . . that masked thing like a monkey" (58). Jekyll/Hyde's desire to stay in hiding, his appearance as if masked, announces an essential connection between secrecy and sexuality, conspiracy and perverse activity. Furthermore, Poole's inability to identify the "thing" in the laboratory as other than "not-Jekyll" suggests that Hyde cannot be classified, he has no place in the order and history of things.

Hyde is the disappearance of Jekyll. Twice in his correspondence Jekyll refers to the event of his "death or disappearance." The first reference to this occurrence comes in Jekyll's will. He writes: "[I]n case of Dr. Jekyll's 'disappearance or unexplained absence for any period exceeding three calendar months' the said Edward Hyde should step into the said Henry Jekyll's shoes without further delay" (10–11). The second reference is written upon Lanyon's last testament addressed to Utterson and not to be opened "until the death or disappearance of Dr. H. Jekyll" (44). On this occasion Utterson remarks, "Here again were the idea of disappearance and the name of Henry Jekyll bracketed" (44). The "bracketing" of Jekyll and disappearance makes Hyde a kind of surface effect, an appearance that marks the loss of Jekyll. Although Hyde hides within Jekyll, Jekyll is hidden behind the mask of Hyde and the difference is crucial to the staking out of their particular identities. Hyde is an eruption which disfigures and disappears Jekyll and Jekyll is the reimposition of order which silences and muffles Hyde, pushing him back into, supposedly, the dark recesses of the self. Hyde is hidden but also hides, his secrecy and need for refuge suggest a criminality that inheres to his lack of place. Jekyll, since he is a place, since he has a place, has depth and interiority, the depth of self, the interiority of conscience, and both are flattened by the appearance of Hyde, of what should have remained hidden.

Having and hiding a secret self, then, ensures Jekyll's downfall. As much as the secrecy of hiding Hyde has to do with a Victorian conception of self and identity, it has everything to do with sexuality. In an essay that links Stevenson's novel to the "new sexology" in the nineteenth century and to the history of perversion, Stephen Heath writes: "Hyde is not just the hidden but also the hide of the beast that he is. The 'animal,' indeed, is Stevenson's cover, what he hides in to write his story: we all have the animal in us (the phylogenetic paradigm) but the animal is a representation of the male sexual which is pathological (perversions, lust-murder)."[18] The animal, Stevenson's cover, according to Heath, unites race — "the phylogenetic paradigm" — with sexuality to explain the threat Hyde poses to Jekyll's body and to bourgeois cultural authority. Unleashing Hyde, Jekyll unlocks the beast of male sexuality and allows it to wreak havoc upon the streets and upon his own body. The apelike Hyde combines perversion with a lust for murder, he allies sex with violence, and he produces within his own person a form and shape for deviant sexuality.

In calling the "animal" a cover for Stevenson, then, Heath refers to the difficulty of representing perversion. Linking *Dr. Jekyll and Mr. Hyde* with Krafft-Ebing's *Psychopathia Sexualis,* published in the same year, Heath shows that the problem in both works was not defining perversion but representing it. Stevenson, he claims, uses the animal image, therefore, to represent perverse sexuality in terms of a primitive and atavistic desire that reduces man once more to the status of animal. But, as I suggested earlier, representation is also a means of producing otherness as sexual otherness. Indeed, Sander Gilman has claimed that "perversion is the basic quality ascribed to the sexuality of the Other."[19]

We can link the perverse sexuality of the other with the medicalization of sexuality as described by Michel Foucault. Figuring power and pleasure as a dynamic spiral, a relationship between surveillance and perversion, Foucault understands the medicalization of sex as both a restraint on sexuality and a production of perverse sexualities. Hyde's relation to Jekyll, in fact, depicts very nicely the spiral of power and pleasure identified by Foucault within the medicalization of sex. If Jekyll represents power, bourgeois power, Hyde represents the pleasure denied and yet produced by the bourgeois subject. Hyde is repressed, hidden, and yet he springs forth from the very body, the very desires of the respectable Jekyll. By conjuring Hyde up from the mysterious recesses of his own desires, Jekyll forges a relation to his own "perversity" — a sexuality that is onanistic, homoerotic, and sadistic — that imposes perversion upon a set of behaviors that he systematically disassociates from himself. Cursing himself for his secret desires, Jekyll turns to science to find the way to both pleasure and power, indulgence and repression. The doubled subject split between desire and respectability identifies power as the ability to be "radically both."

In *The History of Sexuality* Foucault writes:

> [S]ince sexuality was a medical and medicalizable object, one had to try and detect it — as a lesion, a dysfunction, or a symptom — in the depths of the organism, or on the surface of the skin, or among all the signs of behavior. The power which thus took charge of sexuality set about contacting bodies, caressing them with its eyes, intensifying areas, electrifying surfaces, dramatizing troubled moments. It wrapped the sexual body in its embrace. (44)

Hyde embodies sexuality as perversion and degeneration. Jekyll creates Hyde by drinking the right mixture of chemicals after experimenting long and hard in his medical laboratory. Hyde, quite obviously, then, is a product of medicine, a side effect of chemical experimentation. We can figure Jekyll as the power of medicine which precisely set about "contacting bodies," "intensifying areas," "electrifying surfaces," and "dramatizing troubled moments." He is also, of course, the agent that "wrapped the sexual body in its embrace." For Foucault medicine produces perversion in exactly the process that Jekyll uses to produce Hyde. Jekyll chemically creates a perverse body and then he spends the rest of his life trying to repress it and discipline it.

In *The Picture of Dorian Gray*, perversion is produced precisely as a secret; but in this text it is not a chemical substance that allows it to surface, it is artistic method. The malleability of the portrait of Dorian, its ability to shift and change, allows it to record the secrecy of vice upon its painted surface. Basil Hallward warns Dorian: "Sin is a thing that writes itself across a man's face. It cannot be concealed. People talk of secret vices. There are no such things. If a wretched man has a vice, it shows itself in the lines of his mouth, the droop of his eyelids, and moulding of his hands even" (149–50). Here the secrecy of sin and its revelation is a textual event that takes place upon the body. The body that has sin written upon it of course is a monstrous body and a textual body; it is also a body that has been written. The textual event of monstrosity becomes here another chapter in what Foucault calls "the history of sexuality" and the monster records the place and time that the perverse enters discourse.

How is the doubling of Jekyll and Hyde different from or similar to the doubling of Dorian Gray and his picture? And how or why do we read doubling as a sign of buried sexuality in both stories? In both novels another self is produced through experimentation and that self takes over the original. In Wilde's novel the other self is an outer rather than an inner self, it is hidelike, all surface, a canvas; but unlike Stevenson's Hyde, the portrait exists apart from Dorian Gray. As we noted, while science separated Jekyll from Hyde and seemed to produce a repressed self from a surface self, here art serves to separate Dorian from his hideous other spatially.

Like Hyde, the portrait is defined by its need to be confined, enveloped, hidden. Dorian, indeed, keeps it almost perpetually under wraps and finally stores it away in an attic or closet—the portrait is "monstrous and loathsome," a thing to be "hidden away in a locked room" (121). Like Hyde, the portrait must be housed somewhere secret—Hyde lives in a small apartment in the back alley behind Jekyll's respectable mansion, the portrait is banished to an attic room. The rooms become closets but they also represent the relation between self and other as the relation between house and inhabitant—Hyde lives in Jekyll, the portrait lives in Dorian's home. The small closeted spaces also seem to represent on some level the unconscious, a dark space into which forbidden desires are repressed.

Jekyll describes Hyde as "knit closer to him than a wife" (101) and envisions the opposition between himself and his double in terms of the animal versus the spiritual. The relation between the two characters, then, is made explicitly sexual, a parody of both the maternal (Jekyll carries Hyde within him) and the marital relation ("knit closer to him than a wife") and it is explained as a primitive condition of the self. The (male) individual, in other words, carries within himself the germ of a primitive and animalistic sexuality which must be repressed for fear of endangering the very moral fabric of civilization; hence, as Foucault suggests, one had to try to detect sexuality "as a lesion, a dysfunction, a symptom — in the depths of the organism or on the surface of the skin. . . ."

But the sexuality that animates the bond between Jekyll and his double and between Gray and his painting is not amorphously perverse. It is, as we have noted, specifically homoerotic. Secret selves, in Gothic, denote sexual secrets, secrets of the closet more often than not. Certainly in *The Picture of Dorian Gray* and *Dr. Jekyll and Mr. Hyde,* the Gothic monstrosity of Dorian and definitely of Mr. Hyde have everything to do with the sexual secrets that they represent. We cannot therefore explain the monstrosity of a Hyde or a Dorian Gray by saying that they embody sexual secrets, rather we must say that each figure creates secrecy as the precondition for sexual perversity.

Many studies of *Dr. Jekyll and Mr. Hyde* comment upon the device of doubling as a way of representing Hyde as the return of the repressed that disrupts the unity of the self. For example, Gordon Hirsch, in "*Frankenstein*, Detective Fiction and *Jekyll and Hyde*," writes: "The novel's terror, then, comes from the fear of losing control over the parts of the self, from losing any sense of a coherent personal identity. . . ."[20] But of course, this definition of the self as unified proceeds from the specter of its incoherence and not the other way around. Similarly, William Veeder's essay in the same volume, "Children of the Night: Stevenson and Patriarchy," makes male doubles a precondition for patriarchy. However, he explains male doubling or homoerotic desires in terms of "unresolved oedipal complexes" and therefore produces a psychological cause for material effects. I am arguing that, in fact, psychological explanations for human behavior are effects rather than causes of patriarchy. Gothic narratives, in fact, create subjects who produce pathological versions of themselves through extreme self-examinations and they produce, therefore, the sense that individual psyches cause material oppressions. In fact, the monster, as the subject's double, represents not simply that which is buried in the self, rather the monster is evidence of the production of multiformed egos. Indeed, it is only the evidence of one self buried in the other that makes the subject human.

The construction of the doubled subject, one trapped inside the other, is detailed in *Discipline and Punish* by Michel Foucault. Foucault links the emergence of modern subjectivity to the disappearance of torture, public hangings, and all manner of public displays of punishment in the nineteenth century. Such a transformation, he claims, is related to "great institutional transformations" rather than simply indicating the process by which disciplinary measures become "humanized."[21] As public displays subside in the eighteenth century, he claims, "punishment becomes the most hidden part of the penal process" and minds rather than simply bodies become the object of social control: "Physical pain, the pain of the body itself, is no longer the constitutive element of the penalty. From being an art of unbearable sensations punishment has become an economy of suspended rights" (11). The hangman or executioner is then replaced by what Foucault calls "a whole army of technicians: warders, doctors, chaplains, psychiatrists, psychologists, educationalists, etc." We might add lawyers and writers to this list.

If the body is no longer the object of punishment, says Foucault, then something must take its place and that something is the soul: "The soul is the effect and instrument of a political anatomy; the soul is the prison of the body." The novel, as I have suggested elsewhere in this study, is heavily involved in the process by which the soul becomes an "instrument of political anatomy."[22] Gothic novels — because they emphasize and dwell upon the unnatural relations between inside and outside, because they chart the transition of inside to outside, because they turn bodies and minds inside out in their search for monstrosities — Gothic novels play a significant role in the history of discipline and punishment. The Gothic monster is precisely a disciplinary sign, a warning of what may happen if the body is imprisoned by its desires or if the subject is unable to discipline him- or herself fully and successfully. The failure to self-discipline, as exemplified by both Dr. Jekyll and Dorian Gray, results in social death, outcast and outlaw status, and ultimately physical demise. The monster (from *de-monstrare*) encourages readers to read themselves and their own bodies and scan themselves for signs of devolution.

In *The Strange Case of Dr. Jekyll and Mr. Hyde,* Jekyll's strange "case" is not his body but his soul, a soul that divides against itself and becomes its own warder, doctor, educator. Jekyll's body is a disciplined body, a body that understands itself to be in the grips of conscience, under the higher power of discipline. Jekyll produces another self that must be controlled and imprisoned, kept inside; he realizes "the trembling immateriality, the mist like transience, of this so seemingly solid body in which we walk attired" (80). The body clothes the soul but the soul emerges and rules the body: "I bore the stamp of the lower elements in my soul" (81).

In Wilde's *The Picture of Dorian Gray,* the body is obviously enthralled to the soul. Shortly after murdering Basil Hallward, Dorian tells Lord Henry: "The soul is a terrible reality. It can be bought, and sold, and bartered away. It can be poisoned, or made perfect. There is a soul in each one of us, I know it" (215). Dorian's proof, of course, is that his soul has been extracted and transferred to a painting that sits in judgment over him. But Dorian, like Lord Henry, represents a failure of self-discipline and that failure is linked to the fact that his soul is separate from his body.

Without the sense that the soul is buried deep within, the body becomes all surface. Lord Henry characteristically inverts the values of depth and superficiality: "It is only shallow people who do not judge by appearances. The true mystery of the world is the visible, not the invisible" (22). Inversion, indeed, defines much of Lord Henry's speech and it is interesting, therefore, that he provides one of the novel's most careful meditations upon the soul and upon psychology, the science of the soul: "Soul and body, body and soul — how mysterious they were! There was an animalism in the soul, and the body had its moments of spirituality. The senses could refine, and the intellect could degrade. Who could say where the fleshly impulse ceased or the psychical impulse began?" (58). Lord Henry characterizes the attempts to separate mind from matter as psychological: "He began to wonder whether we could ever make psychology so absolute a science that each little spring of life would be revealed to us" (58). Lord Henry precisely does not separate body and mind, surface and depth; he revels in the beauty of the superficial. He is never chastened or shamed, regretful or sorrowed; he never looks for meaning in depth or truth in reality. Lord Henry — the "survivor" in Wilde's novel, the one who gets away with more than murder — Lord Henry survives because he has no conscience, he is not available to discipline.

Like *Dr. Jekyll and Mr. Hyde,* of course, Wilde's novel does attempt to delimit very specifically where the mind or spirit ends and the body begins. But the splitting of Dr. Jekyll into Hyde and the division of Dorian Gray between his youthful perfection and the degenerate painting make tangible first the separation of mind and body and then their absolute inseparability. Dorian Gray sees the painting as equivalent to a reading of his subjective self: "But the picture? What was he to say about that? It held the secret of his life, and told his story. It had taught him to love his own beauty. Would it teach him to loath his own soul? Would he ever look at it again?" (91). Reading and writing the self in both of these Gothic tales makes discourse the place where both the soul (conscience) and its horror (monstrosity) are produced.

The picture, to Dorian, is equivalent to a narrative. Art, the novel tells us, must be unconscious, ideal, remote, not self-conscious, realistic, too close. The picture and Dorian and Gothic style, however, infect by revealing the ugliness, the pain, the violence of identity. In its most perfect form, art would tell no story; in its Gothic form, it tells too many stories. To be art it must have no plot, but its grotesque quality is that its line and shadows, its expression and composition tell of the love of Basil for Dorian, they tell of his abandonment of Sibyl, his adulation of Henry, his sins and misdemeanors. Henry has no story, no secrets, he is like his poisonous book that infects by seducing.

When Dorian shows the picture to Basil in order to taunt him with what has become of his artwork, Basil is shocked by the transformation of his representation of Dorian's ideal form. He sees the effect of separating out soul from body: "He held the light up again to the canvas, and examined it. The surface seemed to be quite undisturbed, and as he had left it. It was from within, apparently, that the foulness and horror had come. Through some strange quickening of inner life the leprosies of sin were slowly eating the thing away. The rotting of a corpse in a watery grave was not so fearful" (157). The painting that once revealed too much of Basil's soul now reveals too much of Dorian's. It does so by giving the illusion of an "inner life" that changes radically the composition of the portrait and creates its monstrous depths. Gothic effect in this passage is achieved by balancing surface against depth and revealing the dissolution of one by the other. Just as Jekyll is being eaten away from within by his Hyde, so the picture of Dorian is consumed internally, parasitically by his foul deeds. The representation here of inner reality suggests that monstrosity is precisely an internal not an external feature. Frankenstein's monster terrified people because of his appearance, Jekyll and Dorian are monstrous because an exterior hides a corrupt self. In each case the bad double is an inversion or an inner version of the outer self but in each model of subjectivity, the depth model seems to give way to one that privileges a version of subjectivity as the shifting ground of various surface effects.

Jekyll shakes the doors of "the fortress of identity" and they give way to reveal that one identity imprisons another. Uncanny effect within *Dr. Jekyll and Mr. Hyde* has everything to do with the idea that one self, Hyde, is housed within another. Hyde describes Jekyll as "my city of refuge" (94) and Jekyll recognizes that, as Hyde, he is "hunted and houseless" (96). By suggesting that identity itself is uncanny, that, indeed, the body resembles a haunted house, Stevenson's novel shows the ideological dangers of trying to separate the haunted from the spook.

In the opening scene of the novel, Utterson and Enfield are out on one of their walks. The streets they pass along are noted for the types of houses which line them. One street, a place of thriving trade during the day, is filled with shop fronts which stand out like "rows of smiling sales women" (3). By contrast to the dingy neighborhood surrounding it, this street shines like a "fire in a forest." Utterson and Enfield notice, however, that the "general cleanliness" of the area is disturbed by "a certain sinister block of building. . . . It was two storeys high; showed no window, nothing but a door on the lower storey and a blind forehead of discolored wall on the upper; and bore in every feature, the marks of prolonged and sordid negligence" (3). The "sinister block of building," of course, turns out to be the refuge of Mr. Hyde. It is the backside of Jekyll's eminently respectable house, a place "which wore a great air of wealth and comfort" (18). By symbolizing the two identities that make up Dr. Jekyll as houses, Stevenson makes a connection between housing and identity, facade and character.

The first chapter of the narrative, then, Enfield's "Story of the Door," establishes Jekyll and Hyde as uncanny in relation to their places of residence. Hyde's door is "blistered and disdained," a place, moreover, where "tramps slouched into the recess" (3). Jekyll's door sits among "ancient, handsome houses, now for the most part decayed from their high estate" (18); while these decaying houses are divided up into "flats and chambers," Jekyll's house alone "was still occupied entire." But Jekyll's house, too, has become a fragmented dwelling as the back door signifies. Between the front entrance and the back exit, furthermore, other divisions mark the space of the home as fractured. When Utterson visits Jekyll, for example, he waits for his friend in a "large, low-roofed, comfortable hall warmed . . . by a bright open fire" (19). This part of the house, however, is divided by an old surgical theater, or "dissecting room," from Jekyll's laboratory. The dissecting room acts as a place of passage between front and back, home and scientific work, the light of bourgeois respectability and the shadow of a criminal underclass. The old surgical theater, one a place for the dissection of human bodies after death in the service of medical knowledge, now signifies the dissection of the living body and the breakdown of holistic identity.

Once Hyde has committed murder and has been identified as a refugee of the law, Jekyll becomes his only hiding place. The game of "hide and seek" mounted earlier by the lawyer Utterson — "If he be Mr. Hyde . . . I shall be Mr. Seek" (15) — now becomes Hyde's mode of existence. Jekyll, as all that remains of the battered "fortress of identity" and of the crumbling stability of home, acts as a place to hide, and a place to Hyde, and the function he performs in housing Hyde produces in Jekyll a murderous anger towards his other self.

In a gruesome parody of pregnancy, Jekyll carries his sleeping, brutal other "caged in his flesh" (101), never knowing when the horror would resume: "[H]e thought of Hyde, for all his energy of life, as of something not only hellish but inorganic. This was the shocking thing; that the slime of the pit seemed to utter cries and voices; that the amorphous dust gesticulated and sinned; that what was dead, and had no shape, should usurp the offices of life" (100). Here, indeed, the house is haunted and the ghost, the "slime of the pit," the hell-baby threatens to consume his host. In suggesting that Jekyll is pregnant with Hyde, Stevenson makes the monstrosity of the Jekyll/Hyde transformation a function of gender inversion and therefore connects bodily duality to sexual difference and a fundamental fear of femininity. The monstrosity, in other words, of a self that hides within one's body is specific to the maternal body, the body deformed and swollen with its other, its hell-baby. Sexual difference within Jekyll's body breaks down and it is the masculine body that swells with the life of another. Since he moves in an almost exclusively masculine world, Jekyll, as divided and dividing, becomes different from his colleagues and friends by becoming woman and alien, feminine and foreign. The combination of sexual and racial difference, as we will see, is crucial to the threat that Jekyll/Hyde poses to the bourgeois order.

The relation between Jekyll and Hyde by the narrative's end, as Hyde threatens to swallow up what remains of Jekyll, is specifically vampiristic. Hyde feeds upon Jekyll, gains from him "his energy of life," and arises from the dead to "usurp the offices of life." The vampire, in Gothic literature, is always an unwelcome guest and the vampiric relation between monster and maker is a part of what we are calling Gothic subjectivity.

The relation between Dorian and his victims is similarly described as vampiric. In one of the most gruesome scenes in the novel, Dorian kills Basil Hallward by cutting his throat. Blood becomes the signifier of criminality throughout this scene. First, Basil attempts to make Dorian pray for forgiveness and quotes Isaiah 1.18 to him: "Though your sins be as scarlet, yet I will make them as white as snow." Dorian, enraged by Basil, "rushed at him, and dug the knife into the great vein that is behind the ear, crushing the man's head down on the table, and stabbing again and again" (158). The body now becomes thinglike: "The thing was still seated in the chair, straining over the table with bowed head, and humped back, and long fantastic arms. Had it not been for the red jagged tear in the neck, and the clotted black pool that was slowly widening on the table, one would have said that the man was simply asleep" (159). Like a vampire, Dorian has torn the man's throat out and let him bleed to death. When he later looks at his portrait he sees "a loathsome red dew that gleamed, wet and glistening, on one of the hands, as though the canvas had sweated blood" (174). Blood, the bodily fluid that marks the inside of the body, also becomes a primary marker of identity in the context of vampirism. As we will see in the next chapter, blood, in Gothic, is always overdetermined — it signifies race as well as sex, gender as well as class and to have blood on your hands is to be implicated in the blurring of essential boundaries of identity. If Hyde lives vampirelike within and upon Jekyll, Jekyll also feeds upon Hyde. And if Dorian lives like a vampire upon the young men whose lives he ruins, they also feed upon him as the abject place of secrecy, sex, and superficiality.

Race and Monstrosity

Henry Jekyll recounts that his discovery of his own dual nature makes him all too aware of the "trembling immateriality, the mist like transience, of this seemingly so solid body" (80). If we want to disrupt the notion that the hidden selves of Jekyll and Dorian Gray are not simply representations of repressed psychic other, it is worth considering what kinds of monstrosity are concealed by only concentrating on sexual or psychosexual monstrosity. Jekyll's hidden self is supposed to represent the base material of his nature, the worst potential of his character. The otherness that Mr. Hyde represents is a composite of a range of alternative identities, identities that literally subvert (overturn from below) the unity of the self. Hyde's deformity depends at least partly upon racist conceptions of the degeneration of the species.

Critics have considered *Dr. Jekyll and Mr. Hyde* as an allegorical treatment of Victorian preoccupations with the instability of body and mind. Such preoccupations arose out of a popular concern with infectious diseases such as syphilis and tuberculosis (which Stevenson suffered from) and a post-Darwinian fear that evolution may be reversible, that, indeed, degeneration was both the symptom and the illness of the age. Race-thinking in the second half of the nineteenth century attempted to allay fears about degeneration and infection by establishing what Hannah Arendt has called "a natural aristocracy"[23] based upon racial purity. As race-thinking gave way to full-fledged racism towards the turn of the century, the body became the setting for a drama of blood. Issues of inheritance, in other words, no longer solely focused on class but now came to rest upon biology and upon the racial body; and predisposition to diseases like syphilis or to the possibility of degeneration were ascribed to certain races (such as the Jews), to their genealogy and their lifestyles, in order to give moral structure to the seemingly random process of infection (Nordau, 1895).

In an essay on film versions of the Jekyll and Hyde story, Virginia Wright Wexman notes that the cinematic depiction of Mr. Hyde very often produces a figure whose repulsion rests upon "racial overtones." Rouben Mamoulian's version of *Dr. Jekyll and Mr. Hyde,* released in 1932, Wexman writes, conceives of Hyde as "a primitive man" and "builds on a racial Darwinian undercurrent in Stevenson's story."[24] Jekyll's evil side, then, as represented by the dwarfish, dark, hirsute Hyde, maps the ugly onto the uncivilized and the evil onto the racially mixed. By making an essential and visual connection between race and character, the film and the novel suggest that human nature depends upon blood rather than circumstance and they both subscribe to a sense of history as a series of fatalities. Indeed, in the nineteenth century, as writers sought general answers to the specific questions of history, Gothic writings contributed to a desire to pin politics, sexuality, and their separation onto biology. For this reason Gothic becomes the place where we can most easily chart the conversion of class differences and racial differences and gender differences into a more neutral category of psychological difference; Gothic, in other words, tracks the transformation of struggles within the body politic to local struggles within individual bodies. The Gothic monster, moreover, as a creature of mixed blood, breaks down the very categories that constitute class, sexual, and racial difference.

The idea of dividing world history into struggles between black, yellow, red, and white races was elaborated in the most detail by Count Arthur de Gobineau in *Essai Sur L'Inegalites des Races Humaines* (1853). Gobineau, a "social pessimist" who predicted the inevitable decline of civilization, believed that civilization was corrupted by the mixture of races and that, while racial purity was desirable, the races were already too mixed and the decline of the species and culture was now inevitable. Defining degeneracy, Gobineau writes: "The word *degenerate* when applied to a people means . . . that this people has no longer the same intrinsic value as it had before, because it has no longer the same blood in its veins, continual adulterations having gradually affected the quality of blood."[25] The popularity of Gobineau's particular brand of race-thinking at a time when many books appeared on the subject may be attributed to his forceful polemic. Hannah Arendt notes: "Nobody before Gobineau thought of finding one single reason, one single force according to which civilization always and everywhere rises and falls" (171). The very specificity, in other words, of the *Essai* marks it as an ideological tool, a foundation for later racisms. Furthermore, by making race the key to historical determinism, Gobineau highlights the body as "the battlefield of history" (Arendt, 175) and suggests that struggle within the individual is historical struggle.

Although Gobineau's writings were not anti-Semitic or overtly racist, they did give rise to racist conceptions of essentially pure and impure races. As the division between races became polarized into an opposition between Aryan and Semitic, or light and dark, the light races were increasingly identified with purity and spirituality while the dark races became the representatives of corruption, decay, and materiality or sensuality.[26] Fields as diverse as anthropology, linguistics, and comparative anatomy participated in ratifying race as "the new key to history" (Arendt, 170). The reemergence of Gothic monstrosity at the end of the century coincides suggestively with the Gothic interdisciplinary interest in the racial body; indeed, by the turn of the century, the Gothic horror novel, from the popular "penny dreadfuls" and "shilling shockers" to canonized works of literature, became a privileged site in the representation of potential dangers of racial decline. The battle for dominance between Dr. Jekyll and his other self, Mr. Hyde, suggests Gobineau's warring races within one body and produces a monster out of the threat that a wave of immigration in London in the 1880s posed to the concept of national character. Indeed, Stevenson depicts the body in this novel as no more than a casing for struggling identities. If Jekyll represents, therefore, the bourgeois individual, Hyde combines within his repulsive aspect the traces of nineteenth-century stereotypes of both Semitic and black physiognomies.

If, on account of its racial content, we read Stevenson's narrative as, at least in part, a text preoccupied with what Homi Bhabha has called the "colonial margin," we can better formulate the disciplinary role of Gothic within a nineteenth-century discourse on race. Race, Arendt has argued convincingly, substituted for nation at the turn of the century as imperialist expansionists attempted to justify their domination of other lands and other peoples. In other words, as the nation expanded to become empire, as Englishmen left the country to go to the colonies, and as a flood of immigrants entered England from Eastern Europe and Russia, national identity came increasingly to depend upon race rather than place. The "colonial margin," in Bhabha's conception of racial difference, as "that limit where the West must face a peculiarly displaced and decentered image of itself 'in double duty bound,' at once a civilizing mission and a violent subjugating force,"[27] describes perfectly the relation between Dr. Jekyll and his hideous double, Mr. Hyde.

Hyde, as the dark side of Jekyll, functions within the novel as a stereotype of otherness. In other words, he embodies the traits of the ugly and the undesirable and makes those traits essential signifiers of evil. In "The Other Question: Difference, Discrimination and the Discourse of Colonialism," Bhabha theorizes the "ambivalent mode of knowledge and power" contained by the stereotype (149). The stereotype, he claims, both fixes the other within racist discourse and recognizes the other as a danger and threat to all notions of origination and racial purity. The ambivalent aspect of the stereotype is, then, a function of the possible simultaneity of fear and desire within representations of otherness, a possibility that may be understood according to "the Freudian fable of fetishism" (160). Within this fable recognition and disavowal of castration allow the subject to maintain contradictory beliefs about an originary sexual difference; difference, in other words, is both acknowledged and subsumed in a process which reestablishes a sense of totality, wholeness, and similarity. Bhabha's proposal that colonial discourse creates stereotypes as fetishes allows him to discuss colonialism as a discipline, as, in other words, a "non-repressive form of knowledge" which can sustain opposing views and contradictions. I find Bhabha's formulation to be very helpful in thinking about the productive nature of othering and the way othering always constructs selves precisely because

Bhabha, in his use of psychoanalysis, manages to avoid reducing all social and political difference to a psychological mechanism. Rather, Bhabha allows us to comprehend the ways in which social and political antipathies are constructed through and as psychic mechanisms.[28] He sees psychoanalysis as not only an explanation of the psyche of domination and submission but also as a description of what Foucault calls "the implantation of perversions" in *The History of Sexuality,* vol. 1.

If the fetish is a "penis-substitute," in Freud's words, "a substitute for the woman's (mother's) phallus which the little boy once believed in and does not want to forego,"[29] the stereotype is a kind of skin substitute which glosses over racial difference and yet maintains it as otherness. That is to say, race and sex both circulate within the economy of the fetish. Bhabha shows convincingly that racial and sexual differences are denied by the stereotype-fetish or the "stereotype-as-suture" (167) although the threatening aspect of both, "the threatened return of the look" (169) is maintained. Again, the importance of this formulation lies in its ability to show the complex structure of racial stereotyping in relation to the various mechanisms of sexual stereotyping.

Hyde is the fetish figure that Jekyll both recognizes and disavows. His appearance inspires hatred in all who observe him, although no one can precisely say what is so repulsive about him. Utterson remarks: "He is not easy to describe. There is something wrong with his appearance; something displeasing, something down-right detestable. I never saw a man I so disliked, and yet I scarce know why. He must be deformed somewhere" (8). Deformity, we are told, inheres to Hyde; his face carries "Satan's signature" upon it, his body suggests "something troglodytic" (18). As a stereotype of otherness, Hyde must represent the not-human; as a fetish figure within the novel, he hides a lack, a generalized anxiety about identity (national and individual).

The essential splitting of the self that occurs in Jekyll's transformation into Hyde makes explicit the duality of the stereotype. Jekyll is quite literally sutured to Hyde and ever in danger of slippage back into the dangerous other persona. In allegorizing the potentially fragmented nature of a certain kind of subjectivity (the other's), Stevenson's novel both assures readers of the possibility of wholeness and yet confronts them with the fragility of the whole. Jekyll/Hyde may be split and splitting but Utterson is an "utter one," a total subject against whom the stereotype, the dark and evil other, cannot prevail. Hyde, then, is stereotyped in this novel by his physiognomy and by his essential role as other to

Jekyll's self. Small, dark, and ugly, Hyde manifests the evil side of Jekyll in a physical form that marks vice upon the body and makes an essential connection between sin and hideous aspect. The body, in this novel, represents the aesthetic space in which sexuality and race conspire to determine human destinies. Hyde as a racial stereotype fixes sexual and racial difference within a body which combines horrific effect with Semitic and Negroid features.

Hyde's name, as we have discussed, puns skin — "hide" — with secrecy and it is within this pun that the relation between race and sexuality becomes clear. While the sexual fetish remains a sign of the difference that must be kept secret, the skin, and specifically skin color, is difference that cannot be hidden. Secret and perverse motivations, then, the sexuality of the other, are announced by the ugliness of the outward appearance; sexuality and race, desire and blood, work in tandem to define otherness. Bhabha again explains this relation within racist discourse: "First, the schema of colonial discourse — what Fanon calls the epidermal schema — is not, like the sexual fetish, a secret. Skin as the key signifier of cultural and racial difference in the stereotype, is the most visible of fetishes, recognized as common knowledge in a range of cultural, political, historical discourses" (166). Here again, the fetish does not summarize racial discourse or displace it into the realm of the sexual; the fetish reveals the multilayered process of stereotyping which functions through many different axes of representation. Racial stereotyping occurs metonymically and at the surface; sexual stereotyping occurs metaphorically and as a secret. Furthermore, the surfacing of one layer of the stereotype eclipses the other and therefore obscures the dual or multiple functions of othering.

Hyde is both a sexual secret, the secret of Jekyll's undignified desires, and a visible representation of physical otherness. The fact that observers can describe Hyde's appearance — he is "small," "dwarfish," "ape-like," "troglodytic," a "masked thing like a monkey" — but cannot say what it is about him that gives such a strong impression of deformity suggests that evil is both the most visible and the most invisible of traits. Jekyll's double has deformity hidden within him and blatantly inscribed upon his hide, his skin. Hyde's doubleness, then, the pun of his name and the relation between himself and Jekyll, represents difference as always a function of both race and sexuality.

Hyde's monstrosity, his hideous aspect and his perverse desires, transforms the politics of race into a psychological struggle between competing identities within one body. By reading the metamorphosis of a Jekyll into a Hyde in terms of Bhabha's "colonial margin," we find that racial and sexual otherness are not hidden within respectability, they are produced by it. Keeping in mind Michel Foucault's analysis of Victorian sexuality as not a repressive system but, in fact, a "proliferation of discourses" (18), *Dr. Jekyll and Mr. Hyde* contributes to a history of sexuality which generates otherness (in this case racial otherness) alongside bourgeois morality.

While the racial discourse produced by *Dr. Jekyll and Mr. Hyde* is not so obvious in relation to Dorian Gray's monstrosity, there is nonetheless a figure in *The Picture of Dorian Gray* who is described as monstrous, and precisely in racial terms. Dorian is telling Lord Henry about his visit to the theater where he saw and fell in love with Sybil Vane. At the theater he encounters a monster: "A hideous Jew, in the most amazing waistcoat I ever beheld in my life, was standing at the entrance, smoking a vile cigar. He had greasy ringlets, and an enormous diamond blazed in the center of a soiled shirt. 'Have a box, my Lord?' he said, when he saw me, and he took off his hat with an air of gorgeous civility. There was something about him, Harry, that amused me. He was such a monster" (48). This monster, the Jew, charges Dorian a guinea for his seat and then tries to find out if Dorian is a drama critic or publicist. He is naturally disappointed to find out that Dorian is merely a lover of the theater and he tells Dorian that theater critics are in a conspiracy against him. Dorian concludes his harangue about the Jew by noting: "He was a most offensive brute, though he had an extraordinary passion for Shakespeare" (52).

What are we to make of the appearance of this other monster in the monstrous tale of Gothic production? It is not enough to point to the anti-Semitism of this scene, of course; rather, what is notable about the anti-Semitic depiction of "the horrid old Jew" (52) is that the Jew's monstrosity is precisely a function of the same characteristics that mark Dorian as monstrous. The Jew is a parasite upon art, according to the text; he makes his living from the theater, he has pecuniary interests in whether Dorian might be a theater critic, and he sells theater for a profit. Art for anything but art's sake, art as functional, is punishable in this text. Dorian uses art to deflect his own corruption and Basil uses art to hide or expose his love for Dorian. The Jew uses art to make a living and therefore is as corrupt as the others. But also, like Dorian, like the aesthetes and dandies, the Jew is depicted as parasitical in his inability to produce anything original. He is not an artist using art, he is merely a business-man who lives off the success of other people's art.

The monster Jew is a substitute for the multiple monstrosities of Dorian and his dandies. He condenses, in one supposedly repulsive form, the economic and aesthetic violations that add up to monstrosity. He, like Dorian, is not an original (the portrait is the real original now) and he becomes another Gothic surface to reflect the breakdown of authentic and artistic subjecthood into an army of imitations.

Conclusion

Dr. Jekyll and Mr. Hyde was discontinued as a theater production in 1892 when Jack the Ripper stalked the streets of London. Critics felt it was inappropriate to entertain audiences with images that resonated with the all too real terror of the Ripper. *The Picture of Dorian Gray* was used as evidence for the prosecution in the trial of Oscar Wilde on charges of homosexual activity in 1895. In both cases life and art came into conflict and the text threatened to merge with the real. Monsters, indeed, tend to blur the distance between the real and the imagined; they set a fragile limit on the powers of representation and they force us to consider the difference between real violence committed upon monsters by "justice" (as in the trial of Oscar Wilde) and literary violence com-mitted by monsters upon respectable citizens (as in Hyde's brutal mur-der of the old man). The link between a Jack the Ripper and a Mr. Hyde, a Dorian Gray and an Oscar Wilde is unclear; the relation between repre-sentations and reality in these cases is what we might now call "Gothic." It is negotiable, shifting, and unpredictable but usually monstrous.

I have been using the term "Gothic" throughout to attempt to iden-tify the moment in writing when interpretation becomes monstrous, spawns monsters, and fixes othernesses in highly specific sites. The ease with which the monstrous form can take the imprint of race or sexuality, of class or gender, as we saw in relation to *Frankenstein,* suggests that Gothic form is precisely designed for the purposes of multiple interpre-tations. We can read homophobic and racist discourses running through the body of the monster and we can as easily find traces of sexist or classist constructions of subjectivities. What we should resist at all costs, therefore, is the impulse to make the monster stabilize otherness. What the monster does in the tales of doubled monstrosity that I have exam-ined here is to call into question the project of interpretation that seeks to fix meaning in the body of the monster. The texts are Gothic inasmuch as they make language or representation itself into the place of monstrous affect.

Dorian Gray becomes Lord Henry's clay to mold when he is struck by the power of words: "Words! Mere words! How terrible they were! How clear and vivid, and cruel! One could not escape from them. And yet what a subtle magic there was in them! They seemed to be able to give a plastic form to formless things, and to have a music of their own" (19). The plasticity of words that Dorian remarks upon recalls Robert Louis Stevenson's impression that literary form was "so much plastic material." The word "plastic" in both contexts connotes the Greek sense of *plastikos* meaning "molded." The Gothic text is plastic because it makes monsters out of words and it makes texts out of monsters and it invites readers into a free zone of interpretive mayhem. The pleasure of monsters lies in their ability to mean and to appear to crystallize meaning and give form to the meaning of fear. The danger of monsters lies in their tendency to stabilize bias into bodily form and pass monstrosity off as the obverse of the natural and the human. But monsters are always in motion and they resist the interpretive strategies that attempt to put them in place. And that, as Donna Haraway puts it, is their "promise."[30]

Technologies of Monstrosity:

Bram Stoker's Dracula

Once Bitten Twice Shy

By way of an introduction to Bram Stoker's *Dracula,* I want to tell my own story about being consumed and drained by the vampire. Reading *Dracula* for the first time years ago, I thought I noticed something about vampirism that had been strangely overlooked by critics and readers. Dracula, I thought, with his peculiar physique, his parasitical desires, his aversion to the cross and to all the trappings of Christianity, his blood-sucking attacks, and his avaricious relation to money, resembled stereotypical anti-Semitic nineteenth-century representations of the Jew. Subsequent readings of the novel with attention to the connections in the narrative between blood and gold, race and sex, sexuality and ethnicity confirmed my sense that the anti-Semite's Jew and Stoker's vampire bore more than a family resemblance. The connection I had made began to haunt me. I uncovered biographical material and discovered that Stoker was good friends with, and inspired by, Richard Burton, the author of a tract reviving the blood libel against Jews in Damascus.[1] I read essays by Stoker in which he railed against degenerate writers for not being good Christians.[2] My conclusions seemed sound, the vampire and the Jew were related and monstrosity in the Gothic novel had much to do with the discourse of modern anti-Semitism.

Towards the end of my preliminary research, I came across a fantastic contemporary news piece which reported that the General Mills cereal company was being sued by the Anti-Defamation League because Count Chocula, the children's cereal character, was depicted on one of

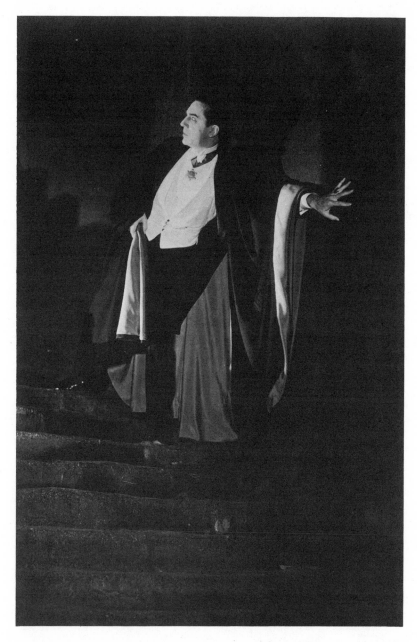

Bela Lugosi as Dracula. In this image, the medallion around Dracula's neck resembles a star of David. This is the image the Count Chocula character is modelled on.

their cereal boxes wearing a Star of David.[3] While I felt that this incident vindicated my comparison between Jew and vampire, doubts began to creep in about stabilizing this relationship. By the time my doubts had been fully expressed and confirmed by other readers, I discovered that, rather than revealing a hidden agenda in Stoker's novel, I had unwittingly essentialized Jewishness. By equating Jew and vampire in a linear way, I had simply stabilized the relationship between the two as a mirroring but had left many questions unanswered, indeed unasked, about the production of monstrosity, whether it be monstrous race, monstrous class, monstrous sex.

Technologies of Monstrosity

Attempts to consume Dracula and vampirism within one interpretive model inevitably produce vampirism. They reproduce, in other words, the very model they claim to have discovered. So, an analysis of the vampire as perverse sexuality runs the risk of merely stabilizing the identity of perversity, its relation to a particular set of traits. The comparison between Jew and vampire still seems interesting and important to me but for different reasons. I am still fascinated by the occlusion of race or ethnicity in critical interpretations of the novel but I am not simply attempting now to bring those hidden facets to light. Instead, I want to ask how the Gothic novel and Gothic monsters in particular produce monstrosity as never unitary but always an aggregate of race, class, and gender. I also want to suggest that the nineteenth-century discourse of anti-Semitism and the myth of the vampire share a kind of Gothic economy in their ability to condense many monstrous traits into one body. In the context of this novel, Dracula is otherness itself, a distilled version of all others produced by and within fictional texts, sexual science, and psychopathology. He is monster and man, feminine and powerful, parasitical and wealthy; he is repulsive and fascinating, he exerts the consummate gaze but is scrutinized in all things, he lives forever but can be killed. Dracula is indeed not simply a monster but a technology of monstrosity.

Technologies of monstrosity are always also technologies of sex. I want to plug monstrosity and gothicization into Foucault's "great surface network" of sexuality "in which the stimulation of bodies, the intensification of pleasures, the incitement to discourse, the formation of special knowledges, the strengthening of controls and resistances are linked to one another in accordance with a few major strategies of knowledge and power."[4] Although Foucault does not talk about the novel as one of these "major strategies of knowledge and power," the Gothic novel in my discussion will represent a privileged field in the network of sexuality. The novel, indeed, is the discursive arena in which identity is constructed as sexual identity; the novel transforms metaphors of otherness into technologies of sex, into machinic texts, in other words, that produce perverse identities.[5]

Foucault identifies the figures of "the hysterical woman, the masturbating child, the Malthusian couple and the perverse adult" (105) as inventions of sex's technology. The vampire Dracula represents all of these figures, he economically condenses their sexual threat into one body, a body that is noticeably feminized, wildly fertile, and seductively perverse. For Dracula is the deviant or the criminal, the other against whom the normal and the lawful, the marriageable and the heterosexual can be known and quantified. Dracula creeps "facedown" along the wall of the very "fortress of identity"; he is the boundary, he is the one who crosses (Trans-sylvania = across the woods), and the one who knows the other side.

But the otherness that Dracula embodies is not timeless or universal, not the opposite of some commonly understood meaning of "the human." The others that Dracula has absorbed and who live on in him take on the historically specific contours of race, class, gender, and sexuality. They are the other side of a national identity that, in the 1890s, coincided with a hegemonic ideal of bourgeois Victorian womanhood. Mina and Lucy, the dark and the fair heroines of Stoker's novel, make Englishness a function of quiet femininity and maternal domesticity. Dracula, accordingly, threatens the stability and, indeed, the naturalness of this equation between middle-class womanhood and national pride by seducing both women with his particularly foreign sexuality.[6]

To claim that Dracula's sexuality is foreign, however, is to already obscure the specific construction of a native sexuality. Lucy, as many critics have noted, is violently punished for her desire for three men and all three eventually participate in a ritual staking of her vampiric body. Mina represents a maternal sexuality as she nurtures and caters to the brave Englishmen who are fighting for her honor and her body. The foreign sexuality that confronts these women, then, depends upon a burgeoning definition of normal versus pathological sexual function which itself depends upon naturalizing the native. It is part of the power of

Dracula that Stoker merges pathological sexuality with foreign aspect and, as we shall see with reference to the insane Renfield, psychopathology. The vampire Dracula, in other words, is a composite of otherness that manifests as the horror essential to dark, foreign, and perverse bodies.

Dracula the text, like Dracula the monster, is multivalenced and generates myriad interpretive narratives — narratives which attempt to classify the threat of the vampire as sexual or psychological, as class bound or gendered. The technology of the vampire's monstrosity, indeed, is intimately connected to the mode of the novel's production. *Dracula* is a veritable writing machine constructed out of diaries, letters, newspaper clippings, and medical case notes. The process of compilation is similarly complex: Mina Harker, as secretary, makes a narrative of the various documents by chronologically ordering them and, where necessary, transcribing notes from a primitive dictaphone. There is a marked sexual energy to the reading and writing of all the contributions to the narrative. Reading, for instance, unites the men and Mina in a safe and mutual bond of disclosure and confidence. After Mina listens to Dr. Seward's phonograph recording of his account of Lucy's death, she assures him: "I have copied out the words on my typewriter, and none other need now hear your heart beat as I did."[7] Seward, in his turn, reads Harker's diary and notes, "after reading his account . . . I was prepared to meet a good specimen of manhood" (237). Later, Seward passes by the Harkers' bedroom and on hearing "the click of the typewriter" he concludes, "they were hard at it" (237). Writing and reading, on some level, appear to provide a safe textual alternative to the sexuality of the vampire. They also, of course, produce the vampire as the "truth" of textual labor; he is a threat which must be diffused by discourse.[8]

The novel presents a body of work to which, it is important to note, only certain characters contribute. The narrative episodes are tape recorded, transcribed, added to, edited, and compiled by four characters: Jonathan Harker, Dr. Seward, Mina Harker, and Lucy Westenthal. The control of the narrative by these characters suggests that the textual body, for Stoker, like the bodies of the women of England, must be protected from any corrupting or foreign influence. Van Helsing, Lord Godalming, Quincey Morris, Renfield, and Dracula have only recorded voices in the narrative; at no time do we read their own accounts of events. Three of these men, of course, are foreigners: Van Helsing is Dutch, Quincey Morris is American, and Dracula is East European. Lord Godalming, we assume, has English blood but as an aristocrat, he is of a different class than the novel's narrators. Renfield, of course, has been classified as insane and his subjective existence is always a re-presentation by Dr. Seward.

The activities of reading and writing, then, are crucial in this novel to the establishment of a kind of middle-class hegemony and they are annexed to the productions of sexual subjectivities. Sexuality, however, is revealed in the novel to be mass produced rather than essential to certain kinds of bodies, a completely controlled production of a group of professionals — doctors, psychiatrists, lawyers. Writing, or at least who writes, must be controlled since it represents the deployment of knowledge and power; similarly, reading may need to be authorized and censored, as indeed it is later in the novel when Mina begins to fall under the vampire's influence. The vampire can read Mina's mind and so Mina is barred from reading the English group's plans. Dracula's reading and Mina's reading are here coded as corrupt and dangerous. Similarly, the English men censor Dracula's contaminated opinions out of the narrative. The vampire, indeed, has no voice, he is read and written by all the other characters in the novel. Dracula's silence in the novel (his only speeches are recorded conversations with Jonathan Harker) is pervasive and almost suffocating and it actually creates the vampire as fetish since, in so much of the narrative, writing takes on a kind of sexual function.

By examining Stoker's novel as a machine-text, then, a text that generates particular subjectivities, we can atomize the totality of the vampire's monstrosity, examine the exact nature of his parasitism, and make an assault upon the naturalness of the sexuality of his enemies. By reading *Dracula* as a technology of monstrosity, I am claiming a kind of productivity for the text, a productivity which leads to numerous avenues of interpretation. But this does not mean that monstrosity in this novel is constantly in motion — every now and then it settles into a distinct form, a proper shape, and in those moments Dracula's features are eminently readable and suggestive. Dracula is likened to "mist," to a "red cloud," to a ghost or a shadow until he is invited into the home at which point he becomes solid and fleshly. As flesh and blood the vampire embodies a particular ethnicity and a peculiar sexuality.

Gothic Anti-Semitism: (1) Degeneracy

Gothic anti-Semitism makes the Jew a monster with bad blood and it defines monstrosity as a mixture of bad blood, unstable gender identity, sexual and economic parasitism, and degeneracy. In this section I want to flesh out my premise that the vampire, as represented by Bram Stoker, bears some relation to the anti-Semite's Jew. If this is so, it tells us nothing about Jews but everything about anti-Semitic discourse, which seems able to transform all threat into the threat embodied by the Jew. The monster Jew produced by nineteenth-century anti-Semitism represents fears about race, class, gender, sexuality, and empire — this figure is indeed gothicized or transformed into an all-purpose monster.

By making a connection between Stoker's Gothic fiction and late-nineteenth-century anti-Semitism, I am not claiming a deliberate and unitary relation between fictional monster and real Jew, rather I am attempting to make an argument about the process of othering. Othering in Gothic fiction scavenges from many discursive fields and makes monsters out of bits and pieces of science and literature. The reason Gothic monsters are overdetermined — which is to say, open to numerous interpretations — is precisely because monsters transform the fragments of otherness into one body. That body is not female, not Jewish, not homosexual but it bears the marks of the constructions of femininity, race, and sexuality.

Dracula, then, resembles the Jew of anti-Semitic discourse in several ways: his appearance, his relation to money/gold, his parasitism, his degeneracy, his impermanence or lack of allegiance to a fatherland, and his femininity. Dracula's physical aspect, his physiognomy, is a particularly clear cipher for the specificity of his ethnic monstrosity. When Jonathan Harker meets the count on his visit to Castle Dracula in Transylvania, he describes Dracula in terms of a "very marked physiognomy." He notes an aquiline nose with "peculiarly arched nostrils," massive eyebrows and "bushy hair," a cruel mouth and "peculiarly sharp white teeth," pale ears which were "extremely pointed at the top," and a general aspect of "extraordinary pallor" (18). This description of Dracula, however, changes at various points in the novel. When he is spotted in London by Jonathan and Mina, Dracula is "a tall thin man with a beaky nose and black moustache and pointed beard" (180). Similarly, the zookeeper whose wolf disappears after Dracula's visit to the zoological gardens describes the count as "a tall thin chap with a 'ook nose and a pointed beard" (145). Most descriptions include Dracula's hard, cold look and his red eyes.

Visually, the connection between Dracula and other fictional Jews is quite strong. For example, George Du Maurier's Svengali, the Jewish hypnotist, is depicted as "a stick, haunting, long, lean, uncanny, black spider-cat" with brown teeth and matted hair and, of course, incredibly piercing eyes. Fagin, the notorious villain of Charles Dickens's *Oliver Twist,* also has matted hair and a "villainous-looking and repulsive face." While Dracula's hands have "hairs in the center of the palm" and long, pointed nails, Fagin's hand is "a withered old claw." Eduard Drumont, a French National Socialist who, during the 1880s, called for the expulsion of the Jews from France in his newspaper *Libre Parole,* noted the identifying characteristics of the Jew as "the hooked nose, shifty eyes, protruding ears, elongated body, flat feet and moist hands."[9]

Faces and bodies, in fact, mark the other as evil so that he can be recognized and ostracized. Furthermore, the face in the nineteenth century which supposedly expressed Jewishness, "hooked nose, shifty eyes," etc., is also seen to express nineteenth-century criminality and degeneration within the pseudosciences of physiognomy and phrenology.[10] Degeneration and Jewishness, one could therefore conclude (or, indeed, ratify scientifically), were not far apart. Stoker draws upon the relation between degeneration and physiognomy as theorized by Cesare Lombroso and Max Nordau for his portrayal of Dracula.

Towards the end of *Dracula,* as Van Helsing, the Dutch doctor/ lawyer, leads Harker, Lord Godalming, Dr. Seward, and the American, Quincey Morris, in the final pursuit of the vampire, a discussion of criminal types ensues between Van Helsing, Seward, and Harker's wife, Mina. Van Helsing defines Dracula as a criminal with "a child-brain . . . predestinate to crime" (361). As Van Helsing struggles to articulate his ideas in his broken English, he turns to Mina for help. Mina translates for him succinctly and she even adds sources for the theory Van Helsing has advanced: "The Count is a criminal and of criminal type. Nordau and Lombroso would so classify him, and qua criminal he is of imperfectly formed mind" (361). Since Mina, the provincial school teacher, mentions Lombroso and Nordau, we may conclude that their ideas of criminality and degeneracy were familiar to an educated readership rather than specialized medical knowledge. As Mina points out, Lombroso would attribute Dracula's criminal disposition to "an imperfectly formed mind" or, in other words, to what Van Helsing calls a "child-brain." Lombroso noted similarities between the physiognomies of "criminals, savages and apes" and concluded that degenerates were a biological throwback to primitive man.[11]

Criminal anthropology, quite obviously, as it developed in the nineteenth century, focuses upon the visual aspects of pathology. The at-

tempt to catalogue and demonstrate a propensity for degenerative behavior by reading bodies and faces demands that, in racial stereotyping,
stereotypes be visualizable. And racial degeneracy, with its close ties to a
social Darwinist conception of human development, also connects with
sexual degeneracy. In describing the medicalization of sex, Michel Foucault describes a progressive logic in which "perversion-hereditary-
degenerescence"[12] become the basis of nineteenth-century scientific
claims about the danger of undisciplined sexuality. Sexual perversions,
within this chain, arise out of inherited physical weaknesses and they
potentially lead to the decline of future generations. Furthermore, theorizing degenerescence or degeneration as the result of hereditary perversion takes, he claims, the "coherent form of a state-directed racism"
(119).

Elsewhere, Foucault claims that "modern antisemitism developed,
in socialist milieus, out of the theory of degeneracy." And this statement,
surprisingly, occurs during a discussion of vampire novels of the nineteenth century. Foucault is being interviewed by Alain Grosrichard, Guy
Le Gaufey, and Jacques-Alain Miller when the subject of vampires arises
out of a discussion of the nobility and what Foucault calls "the myth of
blood." In relating blood as symbolic object to the development of racial
doctrines of degeneracy and heredity, Foucault suggests that the scientific ideology of race was developed by the Left rather than by Right-
wing fanatics. Lombroso, for example, he points out, "was a man of the
Left." The discussion goes as follows:

> *Le Gaufey:* Couldn't one see a confirmation of what you are saying
> in the nineteenth century vogue for vampire novels, in which the
> aristocracy is always presented as the beast to be destroyed? The
> vampire is always the aristocrat and the savior a bourgeois. . . .
> *Foucault:* In the eighteenth century, rumors were already circulat-
> ing that debauched aristocrats abducted little children to slaughter
> them and regenerate themselves by bathing in their blood. The
> rumours even led to riots.

Le Gaufey again emphasizes that this theme develops as a bourgeois
myth of that class's overthrow of the aristocracy. Foucault responds,
"Modern antisemitism began in that form."[13]

I have described this discussion at length to show how one might
begin to theorize the shift within the Gothic novel that transforms the
threat of the aristocrat into the threat of the degenerate foreigner, the

threat of money into the threat of blood. The bad blood of family, in other words, is replaced by the bad blood of race and the scientific theory of degeneracy produces and explains this transition. While neither Le Gaufey nor Foucault attempts to determine what the role of the Gothic novel was in producing these new categories of identity, I have been arguing that Gothic fiction creates the narrative structure for all kinds of gothicizations across disciplinary and ideological boundaries. Gothic describes a discursive strategy which produces monsters as a kind of temporary but influential response to social, political, and sexual problems. And yet, Gothic, as I have noted, always goes both ways. So, even as Gothic style creates the monster, it calls attention to the plasticity or constructed nature of the monster and, therefore, calls into question all scientific and rational attempts to classify and quantify agents of disorder. Such agents, Gothic literature makes clear, are invented not discovered by science.

Gothic Anti-Semitism: (2) Jewish Bodies/Jewish Neuroses

I am calling modern anti-Semitism "Gothic" because, in its various forms — medical, political, psychological — it, too, unites and therefore produces the threats of capital and revolution, criminality and impotence, sexual power and gender ambiguity, money and mind within an identifiable form, the body of the Jew. In *The Jew's Body,* Sander Gilman demonstrates how nineteenth-century anti-Semitism replaced religious anti-Judaism with this pseudoscientific construction of the Jewish body as an essentially criminalized and pathologized body. He writes:

> The very analysis of the nature of the Jewish body, in the broader culture or within the culture of medicine, has always been linked to establishing the difference (and dangerousness) of the Jew. This scientific vision of parallel and unequal "races" is part of the polygenetic argument about the definition of "race" within the scientific culture of the eighteenth century. In the nineteenth century it is more strongly linked to the idea that some "races" are inherently weaker, "degenerate," more at risk for diseases than others.[14]

In *Dracula* vampires are precisely a race and a family that weakens the stock of Englishness by passing on degeneracy and the disease of blood lust. Dracula, as a monster/master parasite, feeds upon English wealth and health. He sucks blood and drains resources, he always eats out.

Jonathan Harker describes the horror of finding the vampire sated in his coffin after a good night's feed:

> [T]he cheeks were fuller, and the white skin seemed ruby-red underneath; the mouth was redder than ever, for on the lips were gouts of fresh blood, which trickled from the corners of the mouth and ran over the chin and neck. Even the deep, burning eyes seemed set amongst the swollen flesh, for the lids and pouches underneath were bloated. It seemed as if the whole awful creature were simply gorged with blood. He lay like a filthy leech, exhausted with his repletion. (54)

The health of the vampire, of course, his full cheeks and glowing skin, comes at the expense of the women and children he has vamped. Harker is disgusted not simply by the spectacle of the vampire but also by the thought that when the count arrives in England he will want to "satiate his lust for blood, and create a new and ever-widening circle of semidemons to batten on the helpless" (54). At this juncture Harker picks up a shovel and attempts to beat the vampire/monster into pulp. The fear of a mob of parasites feeding upon the social body drives Harker to violence because the parasite represents the idle and dependent other, an organism that lives to feed and feeds to live.[15]

Dracula is surrounded by the odor of awful decay as though, as Harker puts it, "corruption had become itself corrupt" (265). When Harker and his band of friends break into Carfax, Dracula's London home, they are all nauseated by a smell "composed of all the ills of mortality and with the pungent, acrid smell of blood" (265). Similarly, a worker who delivered Dracula's coffins to Carfax tells Seward: "That 'ere 'ouse guvnor is the rummiest I ever was in. Blyme! . . . the place was that neglected that yer might 'ave smelled ole Jerusalem in it" (240). The worker is quite specific here, to him the smell is a Jewish smell. Like the diseases attributed to the Jews as a race, bodily odors, people assumed, just clung to them and marked them out as different and, indeed, repugnant objects of pollution.[16]

Parasitism was linked specifically to Jewishness in the 1890s via a number of discourses. In business practices in London's East End, Jews were vilified as "middlemen" who lived off the physical labor of English working-class bodies.[17] Jews were also linked to the spread of syphilis, to the pseudoscientific discourse of degeneration, and to an inherent criminality that could be verified by phrenological experiments. The Jewish body, in other words, was constructed as parasite, as the difference within, as unhealthy dependence, as a corruption of spirit that reveals itself upon the flesh. Obviously, the repugnant, horror-generating, disease-riddled body of the vampire bears great resemblance to the anti-Semite's "Jewish body" described by Gilman as a construction of the nineteenth-century culture of medicine. But the Jewish body does not only bear the burden of a scientific discussion of "race." In his incarnations as vampire and madman, the Jew also produces race as a psychological category. Race, in other words, may manifest itself as an inherent tendency towards neurosis, hysteria, or other so-called psychological disturbances. While this may seem completely in keeping with the larger motives of nineteenth-century race ideology — the division of humanity into distinct groups — the psychologization of race has, in fact, particularly insidious effects. It obscures the political agenda of racism by masquerading as objective description and by essentializing Jewishness in relation to particular kinds of bodies, behaviors, and sexualities.

Dracula's blood bond with the insane Renfield provides a particularly powerful link between his character, the racial and psychological stereotypes of Jews, and Gothic anti-Semitism. Seward's interactions with the insane Renfield fulfill a strange function in the novel; while, one assumes, Renfield should further demarcate the distance between normal and pathological, in fact, Seward constantly compares himself to his patient. "Am I to take it," ponders Seward, "that I have anything in common with him, so that we are, as it were, to stand together?" (114). Renfield's frequent violent outbursts and his habit of eating insects convinces Seward, temporarily at least, that Renfield's insanity resembles rationality only by chance. Renfield's obsessive behavior involves trapping flies to feed to spiders and spiders to feed to birds. Renfield then consumes the birds. Having observed the development of this activity, Seward decides: "I shall have to invent a new classification for him, and call him a zoophagous (life-eating) maniac; what he desires is to absorb as many lives as he can, and he has laid himself out to achieve it in a cumulative way" (75). "Zoophagous," of course, is a term that may just as easily be applied to Dracula and so, the diagnosis made by Seward on Renfield connects the pathology of one to the other.

In "The Mad Man as Artist: Medicine, History and Degenerate Art," Sander Gilman shows how nineteenth-century sexologists marked the Jews as particularly prone to insanity. Arguing that the race was inherently degenerate and that degeneration was perpetuated by inbreeding, Krafft-Ebing and Charcot, among others, suggested that, in Gilman's words, "Jews go crazy because they act like Jews."[18] We may apply this dictum to *Dracula* with interesting results; Renfield is viewed as crazy when he acts like Dracula (when he feeds upon other lives) and Dracula is implicitly insane because his actions are identical to those that keep Renfield in the asylum. Vampirism and its psychotic form of zoophagy, in Stoker's novel, both make a pathology out of threats to rationality made by means of excessive consumption and its relation to particular social and sexual habits. The asylum and Carfax, therefore, the homes of madman and vampire, sit in the heart of London as disciplinary icons — reminders to the reader of the consequences of overconsumption.

In several of his famous Tuesday lessons at Salpatriere, Dr. Jean-Martin Charcot commented upon the hereditary disposition of the Jews to certain nervous diseases like hysteria. "Jewish families," he remarked during a study of facial paralysis, "furnish us with the finest subjects for the study of hereditary nervous disease."[19] In an article on psychiatric anti-Semitism in France at the turn of the century, Jan Goldstein analyzes interpretations of the Jews within the human sciences to show how supposedly disinterested and objective studies fed upon and into anti-Semitism. Charcot's pronouncements on the Jews and hereditary nervous disease, for example, were often used by anti-Semites to prove the degeneracy of that race. Similarly, Charcot's work on "ambulatory automatism" was used by his student Henry Meige to connect the Jews, via the myth of the wandering Jew, with a particular form of epilepsy which induced prolonged somnambulism in the subject. Goldstein writes: "The restless wanderings of the Jews, [Meige] seemed to say, had not been caused supernaturally, as punishment for their role as Christ-killers, but rather naturally, by their strong propensity to nervous illness. The Jews were not so much an impious people as a constitutionally defective one."[20] The pathology of the Jews, according to anti-Semitism, involved an absence of allegiance to a Fatherland, a propensity for economic opportunism, and therefore, a lack of social morality and, in general, a kind of morbid narcissism or selfishness.

Dracula's need to "consume as many lives as he can," his feminized because non-phallic sexuality, and his ambulism that causes him to wander far from home in search of new blood mark him with all the signs of a Jewish neurosis. Dracula, as the prototype of the wanderer, the "stranger in a strange land," also reflects the way that homelessness or rootlessness was seen to undermine nation. The threat posed by the wanderer within the novel, furthermore, is clearly identified by Stoker as a sexual threat. The nosferatu is not simply a standard reincarnation of Gothic's wandering Jew but rather an undead body, a body that will not rest until it has feasted upon the vital fluids of women and children, drained them of health, and seduced them into a growing legion of perverts and parasites.

In his essay "The Uncanny," Freud writes about the roots of the uncanny in the lack of place.[21] He goes on to reveal the mother's genitalia as a primal uncanny place, a place of lack, a site that generates fear and familiarity. Being buried alive, Freud suggests, appears in fiction as "the most uncanny thing of all" but this fear simply transforms a more pleasurable and familiar fantasy, that of "intra-uterine existence" (151). The uncanny aspect of the vampire, however, is not reducible to an oedipal scene because "home" in the 1890s was precisely an issue resonating with cultural and political implications. Coming or going home, finding a home, was not simply a compulsive return to the womb, it involved nationalist, imperialist, and colonialist enterprises.[22] Dracula, of course, has no home and wants no home; he carries his coffins (his only permanent resting place) with him and nests briefly but fruitfully in populated areas. Home, with its connotations of marriage, monogamy, and community, is precisely what Dracula is in exile from and precisely what would and does kill him in the end.

His enemies seek to entrap and confine him, to keep him in one place separate from the native population. Mina Harker, the epitome, in the novel, of all that is good in woman, tells Seward that they must "rid the earth of this terrible monster" (235) and Van Helsing pronounces Dracula "abhorred by all, a blot in the face of God's sunshine; an arrow in the side of Him who died for man" (251).

Dracula, like the Jew — and the Jew, like the vampire — is not only parasitical upon the community's health and wealth, he is sick, nervous, a representation of the way that an unbalanced mind was supposed to produce behavior at cross-purposes with nation, home, and healthful reproduction. The relation between Renfield and the vampire suggests that vampirism is, itself, a psychological disorder, an addictive activity which, in Renfield's case, can be corrected in the asylum but which, in Dracula's case, requires permanent exile or the permanent confinement of the grave. The equation of vampirism with insanity implies an essential connection between progressive degeneracy, hereditary perversion, and a Gothic science fiction of race.

Gothic Sexuality: The Vampire Sex

Dracula's racial markings are difficult to distinguish from his sexual markings. Critics, indeed, have repeatedly discussed vampiric sexuality to the exclusion of race or the vampire's foreignness as merely a function of his strange sexuality.[23] One critic, Sue-Ellen Case, has attempted to locate the vampire within the tangle of race and sexuality. She is interested in the vampire in the nineteenth century as a lesbian vampire and as a markedly queer and outlawed body. She also connects the blood lust of the vampire to the history of anti-Semitism and she opposes both lesbian and Jew within the vampiric form to a reproductive or maternal sexuality. Case describes the vampire as "the double 'she' in combination with the queer fanged creature. . . . The vampire is the queer in its lesbian mode."[24]

Of course, vampiric sexuality as it appears in *Dracula* has also been described as homoerotic[25] and as heterosexual exogamy.[26] So which is it? Of course it is all of these and more. The vampire is not lesbian, homosexual, or heterosexual; the vampire represents the productions of sexuality itself. The vampire, after all, creates more vampires by engaging in a sexual relation with his victims and he produces vampires who share his specific sexual predilections. So the point really is not to figure out which so-called perverse sexuality Dracula or the vampire in general embodies, rather we should identify the mechanism by which the consuming monster who reproduces his own image comes to represent the construction of sexuality itself.

Vampiric sexuality blends power and femininity within the same body and then marks that body as distinctly alien. Dracula is a perverse and multiple figure because he transforms pure and virginal women into seductresses; he produces sexuality through their willing bodies. Lucy and Mina's transformations stress an urgent sexual appetite; the three women who ambush Harker in the Castle Dracula display similar voracity. Both Lucy and Dracula's women feed upon children. As "nosferatu," buried and yet undead, Lucy walks the heath as the "Bloofer Lady" who lures children to her and then sucks their blood. This act represents the exact reversal of a mother's nurturance. Crouching outside her tomb, Harker and his friends watch horrified as Lucy arrives fresh from the hunt. "With a careless motion," notes Seward, "she flung to the ground, callous as a devil, the child that up to now she had clutched strenuously to her breast, growling over it as a dog growls over a bone" (223).

Lucy is now no longer recognizable as the virginal English woman engaged to marry Lord Godalming and the group takes a certain sexual delight in staking her body, decapitating her, and stuffing her mouth with garlic.[27]

When Mina Harker falls under Dracula's spell, he inverts her maternal impulse, and the woman who, by day, nurtures all the men around her, by night, drinks blood from the bosom of the King Vampire himself: "Her white nightdress was smeared with blood and a thin stream trickled down the man's bare breast which was shown by his torn-open dress" (298). Apart from the obvious reversal of Mina's maternal role, this powerful image feminizes Dracula in relation to his sexuality. It is eminently notable, then, that male, not female, vampires reproduce. Lucy and the three female vampires in Transylvania feed from children but do not create vampire children. Dracula alone reproduces his form.

Dracula, of course, also produces male sexuality in this novel as a composite of virility, good blood, and the desire to reproduce one's own kind. Male sexuality in this respect is a vampiric sexuality (and here I diverge from Case's claim for vampirism as lesbianism). As critics have noted, the birth of an heir at the novel's conclusion, a baby boy named after all the men who fought for his mother's virtue, signifies a culmination of the transfusion scene when all the men give blood to Lucy's depleted body. Dracula has drunk from Lucy and Mina has drunk from Dracula, so paternity by implication is shared and multiple. Little Quincey's many fathers are the happy alternative to the threat of many mothers, all the Bloofer Ladies who might descend upon children at night and suck from them instead of suckling them. Men, not women, within this system reproduce; the female body is rendered nonproductive by its sexuality and the vampiric body is distinguished from the English male bodies by its femininity.

Blood circulates throughout vampiric sexuality as a substitute or metaphor for other bodily fluids (milk, semen) and once again, the leap between bad blood and perverse sexuality, as Case points out, is not hard to make. Dracula's sexuality makes sexuality itself a construction within a signifying chain of class, race, and gender. Gothic sexuality, furthermore, manifests itself as a kind of technology, a productive force which transforms the blood of the native into the lust of the other, and as an economy which unites the threat of the foreign and perverse within a single, monstrous body.

Gothic Economies

A Gothic economy may be described in terms of a thrifty meta-phoricity, one which, rather than simply scapegoating, constructs a monster out of the traits which ideologies of race, class, gender, sexuality, and capital want to disavow. A Gothic economy also complies with what we might call the logic of capitalism, a logic which rationalizes even the most supernatural of images into material images of capitalism itself. To take a remarkable image from *Dracula* as an example, readers may recall the scene in Transylvania at Castle Dracula when Jonathan Harker, searching for a way out, stumbles upon a pile of gold: "The only thing I found was a great heap of gold in one corner — gold of all kinds, Roman, and British, and Austrian, and Hungarian, and Greek and Turk-ish money, covered with a film of dust, as though it had lain long in the ground. None of it that I noticed was less than three hundred years old. There were also chains and ornaments, some jewelled, but all of them old and stained" (49). This image of the dusty and unused gold, coins from many nations, and old unworn jewels immediately connects Dracula to the old money of a corrupt class, to a kind of piracy of nations, and to the worst excesses of the aristocracy. Dracula lets his plundered wealth rot, he does not circulate his capital, he only takes and never spends. Of course, this is exactly the method of his vampirism — Dracula drains but it is the band of English men and Van Helsing who must restore. I call this an instance of Gothic economy because the pile of gold both makes Dracula monstrous in his relation to money and produces an image of monstrous anticapitalism, one distinctly associated with vampirism. Money, the novel suggests, should be used and circulated and vampirism somehow interferes with the natural ebb and flow of currency just as it literally intervenes in the ebbing and flowing of blood.

Marx himself emphasized the Gothic nature of capitalism, its invest-ment in Gothic economies of signification, by deploying the metaphor of the vampire to characterize the capitalist. In *The First International,* Marx writes: "British industry . . . vampire-like, could but live by sucking blood, and children's blood too." The modern world for Marx is peopled with the undead; it is indeed a Gothic world haunted by specters and ruled by the mystical nature of capital. He writes in *Grundrisse:* "Capital posits the permanence of value (to a certain degree) by incarnating itself in fleeting commodities and taking on their form, but at the same time changing them just as constantly. . . . But capital obtains this ability only by constantly sucking in living labour as its soul, vampire-like."[28] While it is fascinating to note the coincidence here between Marx's description of capital and the power of the vampire, it is not enough to say that Marx uses Gothic metaphors. Marx, in fact, is describing an economic system, capitalism, which is positively Gothic in its ability to transform matter into commodity, commodity into value, and value into capitalism. And Gothic capitalism, like the vampire, functions through many different, even contradictory, technologies. Indeed, as Terry Lovell points out in *Consuming Fiction*, capitalism demands contradiction and it predicates a radically split, self-contradictory subject. The capitalist subject is both "a unified subject who inhabits a sober, predictable world and has a stable self-identity" and a self "open to infatuation with the wares of the capitalist market place."[29] The nineteenth-century novel, Lovell claims, "is deeply implicated in this fracture within capitalism's imaginary selves" (16). Obviously, the "imaginary selves" of the vampire and his victims exemplify fractured and contradictory subjectivities. Both vampire and victim are figured repeatedly in desiring relations to both production (as writers and breeders) and consumption (as readers and prey).

Vampirism, Franco Moretti claims, is "an excellent example of the identity of fear and desire."[30] He, too, points to the radical ambivalence embodied within the Gothic novel and to the economy of metaphoricity within Gothic monstrosity. For Moretti, Frankenstein's monster and Dracula are "totalizing" monsters who embody the worker and capital respectively. Dracula is gold brought to life and animated within monopoly capitalism. He is, as we have discussed, dead labor as described by Marx. While Moretti finds Dracula's metaphoric force to be inextricably bound to capital, he acknowledges that desire unravels and then confuses the neat analogy. The vampire represents money, old and new, but he also releases a sexual response that threatens bourgeois culture precisely from below.

As with Frankenstein's monster, Dracula's designs upon civilization are read by his enemies as the desire to father a new race. Harker fears that Dracula will "create a new and ever-widening circle of semi-demons to batten on the helpless" (54). More than simply an economic threat, then, Dracula's attack seems to come from all sides, from above and below; he is money, he is vermin, he is the triumph of capital and the threat of revolution. Harker and his cronies create in Dracula an image of aristocratic tyranny, of corrupt power and privilege, of foreign threat in order to characterize their own cause as just, patriotic, and even revolutionary.

In one interaction between Harker's band of men and the vampire, the Gothic economy that Dracula embodies is forcefully literalized. Having broken into Dracula's house, the men are surprised by Dracula's return. In the interaction that follows, the vampire is turned into the criminal or interloper in his own home. Harker slashes at him with a knife: "A second less and the blade had shorn through his heart. As it was, the point just cut the cloth of his coat, making a wide gap whence a bundle of bank-notes and a stream of gold fell out" (323–24). Dracula is then driven back by Harker, who holds up a crucifix, and forced out of the window but not before "he swept under Harker's arm" in order to grasp "a handful of the money from the floor." Dracula now makes his escape: "Amid the crash and glitter of the falling glass, he tumbled into the flagged area below. Through the sound of the shivering glass I could hear the 'ting' of the gold, as some of the sovereigns fell on the flagging" (324).

This incident is overdetermined to say the least. The creature who lives on a diet of blood bleeds gold when wounded; at a time of critical danger, the vampire grovels upon the floor for money; and then his departure is tracked by the "ting" of the coins that he drops during his flight. Obviously, the metaphoric import of this incident is to make literal the connection between blood and money and to identify Harker's band with a different and more mediated relation to gold. Harker and his cronies *use* money and they use it to protect their women and their country; Dracula hoards gold and he uses it only to attack and seduce.

But there is still more at stake in this scene. A Gothic economy, I suggested, may be identified by the thriftiness of metaphor. So, the image of the vampire bleeding gold connects not only to Dracula's abuses of capital, his avarice with money, and his excessive sexuality, it also identifies Dracula within the racial chain of signification that, as I have shown, links vampirism to anti-Semitic representations of Jewishness. The scene vividly resonates with Shylock's famous speech in *The Merchant of Venice:* "I am a Jew. Hath not a Jew eyes? hath not a Jew hands, organs, dimensions, senses, affections, passions? fed with the same food, hurt with the same weapons, subject to the same diseases . . . if you prick us do we not bleed? if you tickle us do we not laugh? if you poison us do we not die? and if you wrong us shall we not revenge?" (3.1). Bram Stoker was stage manager for the 250 performances of *The Merchant of Venice* in which Henry Irving, his employer, played Shylock and so it is not so strange to find echoes of Shakespeare's quintessential outsider in Stoker's Dracula. But Stoker epitomizes the differences between Dracula and his persecutors in the very terms that Shylock claims as common ground. Dracula's eyes and hands, his sense and passions are patently alien; he does not eat the same food; he is not hurt by the same weapons or infected by the same diseases; and when he is wounded, "pricked," he does not bleed, he sheds gold. In the character of Dracula, Stoker has inverted the Jew's defense into a damning testimony of otherness.[31] The traditional portrayal of the Jew as usurer or banker, as a parasite who uses money to make money, suggests the economic base of anti-Semitism and the relation between the anti-Semite's monster Jew and Dracula. I have shown that the Jew and the vampire, within a certain politics of monstrosity, are both degenerate — they both represent parasitical sexuality and economy, they both unite blood and gold in what is feared to be a conspiracy against nationhood.

We might interpret Moretti's claim that the vampire is "a totalizing monster" in light of the Gothic economy which allows Dracula to literalize an anticapitalist, an exemplary consumer, and the anti-Semite's Jew. With regard to the latter category, Dracula is foreignness itself. Like the Jew, his function within a Gothic economy is to be all difference to all people, his horror cannot and must not be pinned down exactly.

Marx's equation of vampire and capital and Moretti's analysis of Dracula and gold must be questioned in terms of the metaphoricity of the monster. As Moretti rightly points out, in the literature of terror "the metaphor is no longer a metaphor: it is a character as real as the others" (106). Gothic, indeed, charts the transformation of metaphor into body, of fear into form, of narrative into currency. Dracula is (rather than represents) gold — his body bleeds gold, it stinks of corruption, and it circulates within many discourses as a currency of monstrosity. The vampire's sexuality and his power, his erotic and economic attraction, are Gothic in their ability to transform multiple modes of signification into one image, one body, one monster — a totality of horror.

Biting Back

The technology of *Dracula* gothicizes certain bodies by making monstrosity an essential component of a race, a class, or a gender or some hybrid of all of these. I have tried to show that gothicization, while it emerges in its most multiple and overt form in the Gothic novel, is a generic feature of many nineteenth-century human sciences and ideologies. Gothic economies produce monstrous capitalist practice; gothic anti-Semitism fixes all difference in the body of the Jew; and Gothic fiction produces monstrosity as a technology of sexuality, identity, and narrative. But I have also tried to make the case for the productivity of the Gothic fiction. Rather than simply demonizing and making monstrous a unitary other, Gothic is constantly in motion. The appeal of the Gothic text, then, partly lies in its uncanny power to reveal the mechanisms of monster production. The monster, in its otherworldly form, its supernatural shape, wears the traces of its own construction. Like the bolt through the neck of Frankenstein's monster in the modern horror film, the technology of monstrosity is written upon the body. And the artificiality of the monster denaturalizes in turn the humanness of its enemies.[32]

Dracula, in particular, concerns itself with modes of production and consumption, with the proximity of the normal and the pathological, the native and the foreign. Even though, by the end of the novel, the vampire is finally staked, the monster is driven out of England and laid to rest; even though monogamous heterosexuality appears to triumph in the birth of Quincey Harker, the body is as much the son of Dracula as he is of the "little band of men" (400) after whom he is named. Blood has been mixed after all and, like the "mass of material" which tells the story of the vampire but contains "hardly one authentic document," Quincey is hardly the authentic reproduction of his parents. Monster, in fact, merges with man by the novel's end and the boy reincarnates the dead American, Quincey Morris, and the dead vampire, Dracula, as if to ensure that, from now on, Englishness will become, rather than a purity of heritage and lineage or a symbol for national power, nothing more than a lost moment in Gothic history.

5

Reading Counterclockwise:

Paranoid Gothic or Gothic Paranoia?

Paranoia and the Gothic

So far, I have concentrated mainly on literary texts to develop a
Gothic history of the technologies of subject production and the relations between human subjectivity and monstrosity. I have used Freud's
theory of paranoia several times in this study to draw attention to the
mechanics of fear production and to suggest the ways in which fear and
desire seem to be produced simultaneously within the Gothic narrative.
Thus, for example, I discussed Frankenstein's "projection" of his own
desires onto his monster and the subsequent translation of his desire into
fear of the other's desire. Furthermore, Eve Sedgwick has claimed that if
the heroine of the Gothic Romance is "a classic hysteric," the hero of
Gothic monster fiction is "a classic paranoid" (*Gothic,* vi). For Sedgwick
the paranoid hero is locked into a homosocial relation to his feared and
desired double. Shelley's novel becomes, as Sedgwick says, "the tableau
of two men chasing one another across a landscape" (ix).

My object in this chapter is to read Freud's two case histories of
paranoia and to discuss the ways in which psychoanalysis degothicizes
the Gothic tales of mental breakdown. Of course, Freud's case history of
Schreber *is* a Gothic tale of the making of a monster and of the feared
merging of human and monster. However, for Freud, monstrosity must
be erased and normality restored. In his case history of Dr. Schreber,
Freud reduces paranoid fear to deformations of sexuality and gender
rather than see pathological fear as a complex conglomerate of social,

cultural, and political hallucinations. For this reason, when he turns to a case of paranoia in a woman, he uses the sexual model of paranoia that he has developed through his male patient, Schreber, to claim for a universal model of pathological fear. Fear, as we know, is gendered; it is also race specific and class specific and Freud's attempts to make all paranoia into male sexual paranoia represent a streamlining of Gothic affect. Such streamlining reduces the complexities of monstrosity to the twists and turns of male sexuality. If we want to measure the contemporary dominance of psychoanalytic models of fear, we can look at the contemporary horror film, as I do in my final chapters, to see that Gothic monstrosity has become Gothic masculinity and fear is coded as the female response to masculine desire. In this chapter I want to reread the case histories of paranoia in order to unhinge monstrosity from masculine power and fear from feminine victimhood.

In his retelling of Schreber's account of his experience with paranoia, Freud insists that Schreber's illness is motivated by repressed homosexual desire and he ignores all other motivating factors. Freud emphasizes the way paranoia reduces all fear to sexual fear quite clearly in "On the Mechanism of Paranoia":

> The patients whose histories provided the material for this inquiry included both men and women, and varied in race, occupation and social standing. Yet we were astonished to find that in all of these cases a defence against a homosexual wish was clearly recognizable at the very center of the conflict which underlay the disease, and that it was in an attempt to master an unconsciously reinforced current of homosexuality that they had all of them come to grief.[1]

The paranoiac is sick only inasmuch as he represents, in Freud's scheme of things, both the homosexual and the fear of homosexuality. The Gothic hallucinations that accompany his fears force the paranoiac to repudiate his desire for men by expressing a fear of persecution by other men. Like Dr. Frankenstein, the paranoiac both desires male companionship and then feels persecuted by it. Like Mr. Hyde, the paranoiac produces the other within himself and then projects that other out into the external world.

Freud transforms Schreber's monstrous delusions into a canny system of knowledge and compares it many times in the course of his narrative to the universe imagined by psychoanalysis itself. The paranoid projection of one man's reality onto a landscape, in other words, becomes a totalizing fiction of identity and culture. Freud explains the human condition in terms of variations upon the theme of sexual pathology and Schreber describes the human condition in terms of a religious system of meaning that revolves around his own sexual body. I will be comparing here Freud's heroic tale of the male paranoiac to his pathologizing narrative of a female paranoiac. We will note that while male paranoia seems to produce a fantastic tale very similar to the Gothic narratives we have been examining, the female paranoiac tells a rather ordinary story about an all too realistic persecution that bears a great resemblance to some contemporary horror film with its insistence upon the terror produced by the unwanted monstrous gaze at the specifically female body.

Schreber's tale of paranoia sounds extremely heroic through Freud's retelling mostly on account of the comparisons Freud insists upon between his own theories of sexual identity and human subjectivity and Schreber's narrative of persecution. Dr. Daniel Schreber wrote up his experience with fantasies of persecution in an autobiography which Freud uses for his case study. Schreber tells of the onset of hypochondria followed by delusions in which he imagines his body is becoming female. In addition to his perceived transsexual transformation, Schreber believes himself to be in direct communication with God. Schreber thinks that by becoming a woman and submitting to the rays of God he will restore the world to a "lost state of bliss." In his delusional state, Schreber believes himself to be the center of the universe as he gives himself over to his bodily transformation. Freud writes: "He has a feeling that great numbers of 'female nerves' have already passed over into his body, and out of them a new race of men will proceed through a process of direct impregnation by God" (113). It is not hard to find in this passage the echoes of Dr. Frankenstein's venture in solo reproduction and Dr. Van Helsing's charge against Dracula that he was attempting to loose "a new race of devils" upon the world. Schreber's monstrosity, like Dracula's and like Frankenstein's, involves both the desire to reproduce alone and the pathologization of that desire. Freud plays doctor to Schreber's monster.

Freud writes at the end of "On the Mechanism of Paranoia":

Since I neither fear the criticism of others nor shrink from criticizing myself, I have no motive for avoiding the mention of a similarity which may possibly damage our libido theory in the estimation of many of my readers. Schreber's "rays of God," which are made up of

the condensation of the sun's rays, of nerve-fibers, and of sper-
matozoa, are in reality nothing else than a concrete representation
and external projection of libidinal cathexes; and they thus lend his
delusions a striking similarity with our theory. (181)

This is a rather remarkable statement in that Freud displays considerable
defensiveness about the collapse of theory into paranoia and the eleva-
tion of paranoia into theory. Male paranoia, within this reading, becomes a rational defense against the corrupting influence of homosexual
desire and psychoanalytic theory is the triumphant heterosexualizing
theory of human sexuality.

The connection that Freud desires and fears between paranoia and
theory has been noted and utilized by psychoanalytic feminist criticism.
In an essay on Freud's "A Case of Paranoia Running Counter to the
Psychoanalytic Theory of the Disease," Naomi Schor rereads Freud to
construct a model of feminist theory. Schor's essay begins with a quote
from Phillippe Sollers that states, "Paranoia is always masculine or feminine" and indeed Schor seems to agree.[2] But she goes on to suggest that
it is dangerous to gender psychological categories (and indeed to psychologize gender categories) because in doing so, one tends to natural-
ize and essentialize both gender and psychology. Furthermore, within a
psychoanalytic system, feminine models of fear and desire are too often
read as pale imitations of their masculine counterparts. The gendering of
psychological categories not only produces stable gender definitions but
also excludes all other traits and traces of the production of fear from
explanatory accounts. If paranoia is only masculine or feminine, in other
words, then it is not black or Jewish, white or Catholic, proletarian or
aristocratic. If paranoia results from gender, then other forms of fear lose
their specificity.

As I have noted throughout this study, the Gothic monster traditionally or conventionally represents multiple modalities of fear and desire and otherness. The success, indeed, of any given monstrous embodiment depends upon its ability to be multidimensional in terms of the
horror it produces. So, Frankenstein's monster and Dracula are "totalizing monsters," they seem to demonize everything that does not conform
to a very narrow notion of male bourgeois humanity. Similarly, Jekyll/
Hyde and Dorian Gray represent a doubleness that is more than double,
a threat that produces monstrosity precisely at the site of human identity.

In the clinical tale that Freud tells about his monster, Judge Schreber, the monster becomes a unidimensional creature, a monster who can be made human by the intervention of psychoanalysis. In this respect, psychoanalysis becomes the antidote to the Gothic tale — the analyst is Dr. Frankenstein finally able to put his monster to rest, or Dr. Van Helsing exorcising the vampire for good, or Dr. Jekyll finding the right chemical compound to save his soul, or Dorian Gray learning to value something other than art. Judging by the many studies of Gothic that use psychoanalytical methods to tell the truth about the monster, modern criticism would seem to confirm that psychoanalysis is indeed the monster killer. But just as one kind of monster dies, another is always produced.

It is curious, in fact, that critics have so often used psychoanalytic models to study Gothic tales of fear, monstrosity, and desire. As my analysis of nineteenth-century Gothic novels has shown, Gothic narrative technologies deploy otherness as a multilayered body marked by race, class, gender, and sexuality. Only a psychoanalytic model of interpretation insists upon the essential link between psychosexual pathology and monstrosity; the Gothic narrative itself sees monstrosity as infinitely more complex and dense. So, Frankenstein's monster may appear within a psychoanalytic reading to represent, for example, the perverse child of an absent mother and an overbearing father[3] but a reading of the text not bound by the psychoanalytic paradigm yields the specter of class or gender inequities. Similarly, a psychoanalytic reading of Stoker's *Dracula* understands the vampire as orally fixated and as bound to his psychopathological other in the character of the insane Renfield but the novel actually exposes the ways in which madness within modernity is always understood through the vagaries of capitalism. Hence, Renfield and Dracula share not simply a mental illness or an oral addiction but a pathologically inflected propensity for overconsumption. In *The Picture of Dorian Gray*, Gray's homosexuality has been read as an abstruse narcissism but it might better be understood as a particular form of monstrosity that depends upon the closet structure of homoerotic desire. Stevenson, finally, makes a narrative of spoiled humanity into a collation of subtexts about primitivism, racism, and nationalism. Jekyll's double, Mr. Hyde, is precisely civilization's "dis-content."

The merging of fear and desire, as I noted earlier in the chapters on *Frankenstein* and *Dracula*, is a staple of the Gothic narrative. The monster in both of these texts, but also in *Dr. Jekyll and Mr. Hyde* and *The Picture of Dorian Gray*, represents the inversion of something like a human identity. Characters in these novels both fear and desire the monster's monstrosity; on a very general level, they desire it because it releases them from the constraints of an ordered life and they fear it because it reveals the flimsy nature of human identity. Monsters, we have noted, embody threats to dominant forms of culture and they represent such threats as self-division or insidious forms of doubling in order to localize Gothic contests to the body. Psychoanalysis, on some level, represents the triumph of one avenue of interpretation; within psychoanalysis social, cultural, national, and political threats become the psychosexual threat of homosexual desire or inversion.

Freud's interpretations of the cases of paranoia fix definitions of horror within a certain narrative, the narrative of psychosexuality. Fictions about fear which locate monstrosity in social, cultural, political, or national frames of reference are here superseded by the fiction of fear as desire or desire's disorder. If paranoia is simply the fear of one's own "aberrant" or nonheterosexual desires, then the sexual self becomes the place that all difference, all perversity, all monstrosity may be located, diagnosed, and presumably cured. Unfortunately, Freud's attempts to skewer monstrosity to sexual perversion have frequently given rise to a gendered grammar of fear and to often homophobic formulations of perversity and violence. If, however, we are able to separate monstrosity from sexual perversion, this may lead to the possibility of an antihomophobic and anti-essentialist theory of the representation of fear and violence. In the last part of this chapter, I look at Alfred Hitchcock's *The Birds* and argue for feminist readings of fear, desire, and Gothic paranoia.

Male/Paranoid Gothic

Masculine paranoia, or paranoid Gothic, and the theory it comes to resemble produces a monomaniacal system which centers narcissistically upon the male body. Feminine paranoia or Gothic paranoia leads to a politics of fear which finds horror to be figured by, but not isolable to, the female body. If Freud suspects that Schreber's pathological description of the ego sounds very like his own "scientific" analysis, the feminine paranoic's perception of self and sexuality comes not only to resemble closely psychoanalytic feminist criticism but it also gives rise to a feminist reading of Gothic horror.

A distinct difference between the two cases of paranoia that Freud studies may be marked at a formal level. Freud bases Schreber's case history solely upon an autobiographical account that Schreber published about his neurosis. Freud justifies the secondhand account saying that paranoiacs often betray "precisely those things which other neurotics keep hidden as a secret."[4] He continues: "Since paranoiacs cannot be compelled to overcome their internal resistances, and since in any case they only say what they choose to say, it follows that this is precisely a disorder in which a written report or a printed case history can take the place of personal acquaintance with the patient" (104). The female paranoiac's analysis, however, is firsthand; Freud meets with the patient when she is referred to him by her lawyer. The effect of making a written account, an autobiography, the paradigm for masculine and feminine paranoia becomes obvious as Freud elaborates his rules for interpretation. Schreber's written and published account seems to acquire a kind of truth value next to the oral history of Freud's female patient. We recall, furthermore, the opposition between written and oral within a novel like *Dracula;* in this text the British ruling class is made up of readers and writers and the oral culture represented by and as vampiric is ironically swallowed up by a kind of imperial bureaucracy. Similarly, Schreber's writing and then Freud's completely subsume the spoken confession made by the female paranoiac.

At the heart of Schreber's paranoid delusion, we read, lies his firm belief that he is on a mission to redeem mankind through his intimate relation to God. The redemption fantasy, however, requires, Schreber claims, that he be transformed into a woman. While Freud understands Schreber's redemption delusion as typical of the monomania that characterizes the paranoiac regression into narcissism, he is at a loss to explain Schreber's desire to become a woman. The fantasy, Freud claims, is "unusual and in itself bewildering" (114); it must therefore be explained as part of Schreber's persecution complex. Freud uncovers a homosexual bond between Schreber and his persecutors (Flechsig, God, his father, and his brother) to explain both Schreber's "unusual" desire to be transformed into a woman and his redeemer fantasy.

Throughout his interpretation Freud commends Schreber on his ingenuity and style: "At every point in his theory we shall be struck by the astonishing mixture of the platitudinous and the clever, of what has been borrowed and what is original" (118). Similarly, as previously noted, Freud finds a certain blurring between Schreber's conjections on neurosis and sexuality and his own. The effect of Freud's unconcealed admiration may be seen at the level of both narrative form and analytic function. Freud's case history itself becomes an obvious example of the "astonishing mixture of the platitudinous and the clever, of what has been borrowed and what is original." Schreber's and Freud's narratives contaminate each other, delusion and theory, clinical analysis and Gothic tale collide until they are bound inextricably to one another. Freud recognizes the process of entanglement and sometimes he fights it, sometimes he rather calls attention to the tendency of the paranoid and the normal to merge.

Freud's method of translation, however, often seems at odds with the sketch of paranoia he has given us. After calling attention to the many places where paranoia partakes in the normal and vice versa, Freud suddenly takes great pains to distinguish clearly between the pathological and the normal, delusion and reality. For example, after suggesting that Schreber's paranoiac disorder may be homosexually motivated, Freud protects himself from imaginary charges of slander: "We are not making reproaches of any kind against him — whether for having had homosexual impulses or for having endeavored to suppress them. Psychiatrists should take a lesson from this patient, when they see him trying, in spite of his delusions, not to confuse the world of the unconscious with the world of reality" (143). Suddenly, when homosexuality is the issue, the real is not to be confused with delusion, the unconscious must not be allowed to contaminate the real. Schreber, furthermore, according to Freud, is a model for the ability to keep such things separate!

"Paranoia decomposes just as hysteria condenses" (149), Freud writes. This simple statement seems to bring us closer to how we might read paranoia as a pathology, as a style of writing, as a process of contamination. Freud has, as we know, invited comparisons at every level between his own theory and paranoiac delusion — "It remains for the future to decide whether there is more delusion in my theory . . . or more truth in Schreber's delusion" — and we are therefore at liberty to make general remarks about the similarities shared by the theory and the delusion. Paranoia decomposes — the autobiographical account upon which Freud bases his theory of paranoia is reliable, he claims, because paranoiacs tell all, they reveal everything. However, the truth value that Freud assigns to autobiography decomposes within the form itself. The narrating subjects multiply — there is the Schreber after his recovery, the Schreber in the grips of delusion, God speaking through Schreber, Schreber as a woman, and finally, Freud speaking through Schreber's account and remarking upon "the astonishing mixture . . . of what has been borrowed and what is original."

Schreber's idea that "after all it must be very nice to be a woman submitting to the act of copulation" (122), according to Freud, provokes him to construct an entire delusional system to facilitate his desire and protect himself from its implications. These implications for Freud are obviously of a homosexual nature but we might object here to the conflation of homosexual and transsexual fantasies. Schreber's desire is quite clear, he fantasizes being a woman "submitting to the act of copulation" and this is markedly different from the desire to be a man for another male. Within a psychoanalytic model, it seems, paranoia is an overwhelming fear of the feminine that necessitates a systematized defense against identification with a feminine subject position and with female pleasure and homosexual desire. Freud's homophobic conflation of femininity and the desire for male sexual attention confuses even the psychosexual terrain of Schreber's fantasy.

The narrative that Schreber produces out of his paranoid episode resembles closely earlier Gothic tales about vampires and monsters. In his Gothic narrative, his body becomes monstrous by internally taking on the organs and forms of the female body and then by submitting sexually to the rays of God. Furthermore, he accuses various professionals around him of "soul murder" or the absorption of human souls by devil-like men. Obviously soul murder bears a strong resemblance to vampirism. God, Schreber says, comes and speaks to him in a "root language" or a "basic language" which often is transmitted through birds. In response to this Gothic fiction, Freud produces another story; this one insists upon a rational explanation for the hallucinated feminine voluptuousness and transforms the desire to become female into homosexually based feelings of persecution.

Obviously, Dr. Schreber's fantasies of his own transsexuality and God's punishing sexual aggression must be comprehended from a psychosexual perspective. But paranoia always also has a political component to it. In their epic critique of psychoanalysis and "familialism," Gilles Deleuze and Félix Guattari take Freud to task for "flattening-out" Judge Schreber's delirium: "It should be noted that Judge Schreber's destiny was not merely that of being sodomized, while still alive, by the rays from heaven, but also that of being posthumously oedipalized by Freud. From the enormous political, social and historical content of Schreber's delirium, not one word is retained as though the libido did not bother itself with such things. Freud invokes only a sexual argument."[5] The use of the term "flattening-out" here seems important. One of the effects of Freud's interpretation of Schreber's case history is certainly the oedipalization of his narrative but it also consists in an erasure of Gothic affect. The gothicizations of the body that Schreber attests to are far more elaborate than a simple fear of homosexual desire might indicate. Schreber's desire to become a woman could as easily correspond to a nationalistically motivated desire to repopulate the earth with superior beings. Indeed, Schreber talks about the existence of lower and upper gods in heaven; the lower god exists for "dark people" and the upper god for "aryan peoples." When viewed in this context, Schreber's desire to become God's wife and bear his children resembles a protofascist impulse to control reproduction and generate a superior race. As I noted in my chapter on *Dracula*, it is relatively easy to find the traces of anti-Semitic and other fin-de-siècle racisms within the gothicizations of the other.

To return for a moment to the passage I quoted from Deleuze and Guattari, another way in which Freud achieves the "flattening-out" of Schreber's narrative operates through the assumption that the libido, as Deleuze and Guattari put it, does "not bother itself with such things" as social, cultural, or political drives. This limited conception of the libido gives rise to contemporary critiques of psychoanalysis; the libido, after all, is always as much a production of race, class, and nationality as it is a production of sex and gender. The reason, therefore, that psychoanalysis feels inadequate to the interpretive task of reading Gothic narratives is because Gothic narratives assume the manifold nature of the libido while psychoanalysis attempts to condense libido into gender and sex drives.

Deleuze and Guattari keep returning to Schreber in order to illustrate the erasures performed upon history by psychoanalysis. The way psychoanalysis reduces everything to psychopathology, Deleuze and Guattari show, renders history obsolete and forces us to psychologize political outrages rather than comprehend them in relation to historically specific nationalist and social and cultural issues. They summarize oedipalization in relation to paranoia thus:

> The fact remains that Schreber's memoirs are filled with a theory of God's chosen peoples, and with the dangers that face the currently chosen people, the Germans, who are threatened by the Jews, the Catholics, and the Slavs. In his intense metamorphoses and passages, Schreber becomes a pupil of the Jesuits, the burgomaster of a city where the Germans are fighting against the Slavs, and a girl defending Alsace against the French. At last he crosses the Aryan

gradient or threshold to become a Mongol prince. What does this becoming-pupil, burgomaster, girl and Mongol signify? All paranoiac deliriums stir up similar historical, geographic, and racial masses. The error would lie in concluding, for example, that fascists are mere paranoiacs. (89)

Paranoia, in other words, forces the subject to gothicize "others" while attempting to elevate or purify the self. Paranoia is precisely a Gothic mechanism, a production of a demon who represents a multitude of fears. But Deleuze and Guattari's caution is well-taken: "The error would lie in concluding, for example, that fascists are mere paranoiacs." Psychological explanations for racist and nationalist sentiment simultaneously produce the need for psychological cures. If fascism is merely paranoia, then fascism represents a large-scale shared delusion that requires psychoanalytic intervention. Obviously, fascism is a far more complicated object than paranoia can suggest and it certainly cannot be explained using psychoanalytic models of paranoia as the fear of homosexuality. For the fascist, concepts of purity, superiority, and ethnic cleansing are always relayed through gendered and racialized frames of reference.

A recent film enacts the problematic effects of psychologizing political movements. *Schindler's List* (1994), the much acclaimed Holocaust film by Steven Spielberg, precisely transforms the story of genocide into an essential psychodramatic story of human nature. The film focuses upon the experiences of one man, Oskar Schindler, a German industrialist who inadvertently saves Jews from being shipped to concentration camps by having them work for him in his factory. Schindler is depicted as unconsciously heroic because he braves Nazi scorn by constantly looking out for "his Jews." The film compares Schindler to a Nazi counterpart, a man of his own age and class, who treats Jews like animals and embodies the stereotype of the sadistic fascist who takes a sexual pleasure in killing and for whom violence actually replaces sexuality. Within Spielberg's production of the story of Oskar Schindler, the Jews are reduced to no-name masses while the real contest takes place between the German who retains a shred of human feeling and the Nazi who exercises a pathological contempt for humanity through sadistic displays of brutality.

The Holocaust has been variously theorized as "unrepresentable" precisely because traditional narrative forms tend to render intelligible otherwise incomprehensible material.[6] The most successful renditions of the Holocaust to date, therefore, have been abstract and non-narrative films like Claude Lanzmann's *Shoah*. By making the Holocaust into a story—into, moreover, an autobiography of a German—Spielberg capsulizes the Holocaust into a tale of two peoples that can be uncovered merely by telling the tale of two or three individuals. Within the film's humanist logic, each individual carries the trace of the story and each body involved in the story experiences it as a whole. In the story that Spielberg chooses to tell, and that an American public chose to embrace, the good German is a capitalist who offers salvation in the way of economic common sense—the Jews represent a work force that it would be an economic shame to waste. The bad German is a scoundrel who casually wastes lives—and therefore workers—to satisfy his own sadistic ego. Psychology takes over by the end of this holistic narrative when Schindler is shown freeing his Jews at the end of the war and chastising himself for not "saving just one more." His humanity, and indeed his humanism, conquers his business sense in this scene and again the crisis becomes one of human feeling versus economics.

So, what does *Schindler's List* have to do with Schreber and his paranoia? I am trying here to show the danger as well as the power as well as the pleasure associated with psychoanalytic explanations for social, cultural, personal, and political crises. The danger of psychoanalytic explanations which cast the Nazi as paranoiac or sadist, the Jew as masochist or also paranoiac, and the good German as humane and preoccupied with economic as well as physical health, lies in their tendency to reinvest in the humanist world of "monsters and men." Today's monster, furthermore, might be tomorrow's victim and the next day's hero. Psychologically based explanations are thoroughly invested in binaries like health versus sickness, waste versus use, pure versus impure, normal versus perverted. But, of course, these exact oppositions prop up Nazi ideologies of racial and cultural superiority.

The power of psychological explanations of political material also resides in their depiction of the world as divided into good and bad people. It is quite ironic, in fact, that Spielberg would film *Schindler's List* in black and white because the world he depicts, the complicated and overdetermined universe of Nazi bureaucratic violence, is absolutely a black and white world where bad things happen to good people and bad people are easily identifiable as monstrous and where the good are saved, the bad perish, and God smiles down upon his people. As we know, after the Holocaust we cannot, indeed should not, believe in such a world, in such people. And it is not simply making monsters that is at fault here but the idea that monsters and humans are separate entities and always distinguishable.

As we saw in *Frankenstein,* monster and maker are involved in a mutual struggle for existence and both partake in the definitions of monstrosity and humanity that circulate in the text. In *Dr. Jekyll and Mr. Hyde* and *The Picture of Dorian Gray,* the stakes of a tangled human/monster subject are quite clear—in these narratives the two coexist within one body. In *Dracula* the good and the pure men of England identify the monstrosity of the vampire as parasitism with regards to the vampire's racial makeup, its bodily features, its sexual practices, and its use of money or gold. The enterprise of vampire hunting, however, strongly resembles fin-de-siècle Jew-baiting. So what do these entanglements prove? Gothic narrative structures, I have tried to argue throughout this book, are never simply reactionary or progressive; indeed, the very desire to identify genres as purely one thing or the other comes out of a humanist investment in the idea of clarity, identity, and essential natures. Gothic is a narrative strategy that refuses purity and indeed, reveals the suspect ideological stakes of quests for purity. Paranoia, within this description of Gothic structures, is the fear that simultaneously blurs boundaries *and* calls for their resurrection. Paranoia, like Gothic, moves in many directions. Within some scenarios paranoia is a homophobic and irrational protection against the desire for homoeroticism, within others it is the irrational fear of the fear of the other; within some deliria paranoia produces fantasies of nationalistic purity and racial selectivity, within others it defends against the fear of racism. Paranoia, like Gothic, represents both fear and the fear of fear.

Foucault's Pendulum, a theoretical novel by Umberto Eco, demonstrates nicely the circular or Gothic structure of paranoia. In *Foucault's Pendulum* a group of publishers create a fictional plan for world domination and attribute it to a secret masonic order. As the plan expands and becomes more and more intricate, the writers come to the gradual awareness that their fiction all along has been seeping into reality. Finally, of course, fiction and life merge completely and the authors of the masterplan understand that they have participated in a paranoid conspiracy theory of history that always produces proof and plot side by side. Eco writes: "If you feel guilty, you invent a plot, many plots. And to counter them, you have to organize your own plot. But the more you invent enemy plots to exonerate your own lack of understanding, the more you fall in love with them, and you pattern your own on their model."[7] Paranoia, in other words, produces "plots" and these plots (narratives and conspiracies) have a way of creating reality. As much as paranoia, then, is a pathological thought disorder, it is also a description of a subjectivity that filters various fears and desires through an overwhelming belief in both the power and the utter powerlessness of the individual in capitalism. Michel Foucault has theorized the relation between power and the individual in relation to the structure of the panopticon. Such a structure produces the illusion in the individual of being watched without necessitating constant surveillance.

In the capitalist era, according to Foucault, all space must be regulated according to modern concepts of law and order. The problem that such regulation presents is of how to exert more complete and efficient control over a population. In response to the problem of surveillance, Foucault suggests, there emerged a new technology and a new economy of the power to punish. The panopticon represents symbolically the architecture of new economies of discipline and punishment. These new economies had to, first, find a way to bind individual wrongdoing to offense against all society, not just the king; second, use "humane" methods in order to use rather than discard the body of the criminal; third, determine guilt and amounts of punishment through reason, not torture; fourth, individualize sentences and classify, quantify, and calibrate crimes and punishments. Eventually, the new economy of power and discipline led to the individualization of criminality through criminology, the study of crime and the description of criminality as no longer simply a political offense but ultimately as evidence of a psychological disruption or disturbance. Foucault consistently links the criminal and the madman in this study: "The criminal, designated as the enemy of all, whom it is in the interest of all to track down, falls outside the social pact, disqualifies himself as citizen and emerges, bearing within him as it were, a wild fragment of nature; he appears as a villain, a monster, a madman. Perhaps a sick and before long 'abnormal' individual."[8]

The disciplines of psychology, sexology, criminology, as we saw in the chapter on *Dracula,* absolutely participate in the production of monsters upon whom all social ills can be blamed. The panopticon version of disciplinarity produces anonymity alongside individuality and encourages a form of paranoia in the subject. For the paranoiac, we might conclude, the only thing worse than being watched is not being watched. If, in our culture, people cling to conspiracy theories, then it is in order to verify their place in the order of things or to convince themselves that an order of things exists at all.

From *Foucault's Pendulum* to Foucault's panopticon, paranoid plots have a serious political dimension that cannot be satisfactorily explained away with reference to psychoanalysis. "Paranoid Gothic," in my rereading of Freud's case history of Dr. Schreber, names the moral panic that characterizes Freud's attempts to flatten-out a fantastic narrative into a conventional story of oedipal desire. If we turn to the case of paranoia in a woman, we see very quickly that paranoia has a way of always "running counter to the psychoanalytic theory of the disease."

Female/Gothic Paranoia

The dividing line between the normal and the pathological becomes almost seamless in "A Case of Paranoia Running Counter to the Psychoanalytic Theory of the Disease." A woman is referred to Freud by her lawyer after she brings charges against her lover, accusing him of "getting invisible witnesses to photograph them in the act of love-making."[9] Freud notes that the lawyer "was experienced enough to recognize the pathological stamp of this accusation" (97). As the story unfolds, it appears that the woman, who was "attractive" and "of a distinctly feminine type" (97), had been involved with a man who could not marry her "for external reasons." The man argues, persuasively apparently, that social convention should not prevent them from having a relationship nonetheless. In order not to compromise the young woman's social standing, the two lovers meet during the day at the man's apartment. During their lovemaking the woman hears a "a kind of knock or a tick" which the man says comes from a little clock on his writing table. The woman, however, later connects the noise to two strangers she sees on the stairs outside carrying a box and she imagines she has been photographed.

Freud feels troubled by the woman's narrative because, while he characterizes it as paranoid, he can find no evidence of the homosexual fixation which he believes to be an integral part of the neurosis. Torn between abandoning his theory of paranoia and recognizing the woman's experience as an actual event, Freud finds "another way out": "I recollected how often wrong views were taken about psychotic patients simply because they had not been studied carefully enough and had not told enough about themselves" (100). We remember, however, that Freud considered Dr. Schreber's censored autobiography to be perfectly reliable because paranoiacs "betray precisely those things which other neurotics keep hidden as a secret." Already the woman's account is seen to be lacking and it is Freud himself who will fill in her "blanks." He asks her to return for a second visit.

Of course, Freud receives the information he desires upon his patient's return. She reveals the presence of an older woman at work whom she suspects of having an affair with her lover. Freud now easily makes the case for a mother complex and female paranoia seems to conform to the male paradigm. To explain the tick that the woman heard in the apartment, Freud elaborates a metaphoric series — camera, clock, clitoris. He suggests that the woman, engaged in a primal scene fantasy, a fantasy of listening and seeing, occupied the place of her mother within the sexual scene and heard the knocking of her own clitoris, her own desire.

By elaborating the process by which a tick is heard as the noise of a camera shutter and then interpreted first as a clock and finally as a clitoris, we may discover a "technology of sex" which produces femininity in a certain relation to discursive authority and then defines a particular sexuality for the female body. In *The History of Sexuality*, vol. 1, Michel Foucault has written about the role of psychoanalysis in the deployment of sex. He suggests that psychoanalysis is "a mechanism for attaching sexuality to the system of alliance; it assumes an adversary position with respect to the theory of degenerescence; it functions as a differentiating factor in the general technology of sex."[10] Foucault's cogent analysis obviously makes psychoanalysis complicit in the deployment of sex. As Teresa de Lauretis has pointed out, the problem for feminism in Foucault's formulation is that he construes sexuality "not as gendered (as having a male form and a female form) but simply as male."[11] It is Foucault's notion here of "mechanism," however, which permits a feminist application to Freud's theory of paranoia.

Freud describes "the distinctive character of paranoia" itself as "a mechanism by which the symptoms are formed or by which repression is brought about" (161). In Dr. Schreber's case, his delusion of becoming a woman reveals the mechanism of homosexual fixation. In the case of the female paranoiac, homosexual fixation becomes a mechanism within a mechanism, a function related to the metaphorical and mechanical intervention of the noise made by a camera or a clock or a clitoris. Since Foucault describes psychoanalysis as a mechanism and Freud describes paranoia as a mechanism, the tick that the female paranoiac hears in her boyfriend's apartment may prove to be the paradigmatic sound of psychoanalysis itself. At stake, then, in the interpretation of the tick is Freud's universalizable system and the place of the feminine within or without it.

By identifying the click she hears as a camera, the female paranoiac remarkably interprets her position within the social and technological relations circumscribed by a specifically *cinematic* apparatus. In *Alice Doesn't* Teresa de Lauretis describes the position of woman within narrative cinema as the object of the gaze, the subject of the other's desire, the "mythical obstacle, monster of landscape."[12] Stranded somewhere between the gaze and the image, she suggests, feminine identification requires motion between alternate subject positions defined as masculine and feminine. She writes: "The analogy that links identification-with-the-look to masculinity and identification-with-the-image to femininity breaks down precisely when we think of a spectator alternating between the two. Neither one can be abandoned for the other, even for a moment" (143). In the scene in her lover's apartment, Freud's female patient understands her subject position as object or image. The secret tryst she engages in has been established, we are told, in defiance of social convention. By placing herself in opposition to convention, the woman exposes herself to certain kinds of scrutiny. The click of the camera is the materialization of the social mechanism that legislates her desire.

The camera, here, represents a particularly suggestive symbol for the mechanism and technology of paranoia and it demands a close reading. In addition to fixing the kind of feminine identification that de Lauretis describes, the camera may also be evidence of the relation between male and female desire as it appears to the woman. In *The Acoustic Mirror,* Kaja Silverman describes paranoiac projection on the part of the male in psychoanalytic terms as "refusal to be that which evokes unpleasure."[13] By projecting otherness and castration onto the female, Silverman suggests, the male can disavow his own lack: "The male subject responds to this threat of (re)contamination with phobic avoidance — by insisting upon the absoluteness of the boundaries separating male from female" (16). "Projection" for Silverman is a "mechanism" which upholds the male's desire for separation. Again, we must note the exclusively sexual explanation that a psychoanalytic approach confers upon the narrative — here, Silverman equates pleasure only with libidinal responses. "The refusal to be that which evokes unpleasure" could as easily apply to racial or class positions as to gendered or sexualized identities.

However, according to Silverman's theoretical frame, the female patient's fantasized camera and its projective function is precisely an "acoustic mirror," a sound which mirrors the function that the female subject must perform in the construction of male subjectivity.

The fantasy that suggests pathology to the lawyer and Freud may actually be an acute reading of the power of voyeurism, the imaged positionalities of male and female desire within the gaze, and the politics of fear from a female or even protofeminist perspective. Moving from the bedroom to the office of psychoanalysis, the camera is fixed by Freud's analysis into a monomaniacal gaze of a universalizing theory. The single-eyed look that froze the woman's desire and interrupted her pleasure is precisely the gaze of psychoanalysis. The mechanism of paranoia that, in Schreber's case, blurred with Freud's theoretical framework now becomes unitary, focused, uncontaminated. The tick, as Freud interprets it, is firmly grounded within the woman's body as the clitoris. Apart from defining the woman's fear of being watched as pathological, Freud has essentialized femininity as specific to the female body. The woman, in turn, proposes a counternarrative that reads the tick as the sound of the masculine gaze which attempts to freeze feminine sexuality within a voyeuristic frame.

The tick that the woman has heard and identified resists, in fact, the kind of interpretation that Freud employs in his effort to clearly delineate between masculinity and femininity. As a "mechanism", and as part of a larger machinery, the noise is capable of producing excess. In this instance the tick signifies both camera and clitoris. It also, however, signifies clock. The clock lies between the camera (the woman's fear of voyeurism) and the clitoris (Freud's fear of femininity); it is the place where interpretation turns in time — clockwise or counterclockwise. We will recall that the English translation of the case history is "A Case of Paranoia Running *Counter* to the Psychoanalytic Theory of the Disease." The discovery of a homosexual fixation which is so crucial to Freud's need to universalize his theory, turns, as we have seen, upon the translation of the case's central mechanism into either machine/apparatus or body. We suspect, of course, that the mechanism is both machine and body, camera and clitoris, and so the case still runs "counter" to the theory. The clock signifies a different temporality; a time frame both linear and synchronic; a regular progression, like clockwork; and an interrupted and oppositional direction, counterclockwise.

The case of female paranoia that Freud works so hard to interpret through a male model may be used to produce the possibility of counter-readings of fear, desire, and narratives of horror. Female paranoia, as I have been trying to show, manifests itself as an almost rational response to masculinist systems of sex and gender. Furthermore, the female case of paranoia uncannily produces a metaphoric series which represents female fear as a conspiracy of desire (clitoris), time (clock), and the fear of being watched (camera).

The paranoiac defense against infection, the attempt that both Schreber and Freud make to write out the boundaries between male and female, proves to always already be contaminated and in the process of decomposition — "paranoia decomposes," Freud noted scrupulously. Horror, for the masculine paranoiac, lies in not knowing oneself as already diseased and yet finding evidence of infection all around. The power of feminine paranoia, or simply feminist critique, lies in its ability to read lack and disfigurement productively and to exist with loss without nostalgically yearning for wholeness. It also lies in broadening the frames of fear and desire to include a whole host of fear-producing factors and to refuse the essential links between femininity and fear, masculinity and power.

Gothic (Feminist) Paranoia and Horror Film

The mechanism of Gothic paranoia, a fear of being watched that produces both fear and desire in the female body and provokes a male sexual response, corresponds to conventional formulae for visual pleasure in cinema. Laura Mulvey's much cited article "Visual Pleasure and Narrative Cinema" lines up Hollywood cinema with patriarchal productions of femininity. She suggests that women are always to be looked at in classic cinema while men are the bearers of the look.[14] Linda Williams, in "When the Woman Looks," asks what might happen if women returned the gaze and she turns to the modern horror film in order to answer her own question. When the woman looks in the horror film, Williams writes, "the female look — a look given preeminent position in the horror film — shares the male fear of the monster's freakishness, but also recognizes the sense in which this freakishness is similar to her own difference."[15] When the woman looks, in other words, she too becomes monstrous. Williams, obviously, then, is ambivalent about what it means for the woman to look but, we might argue, this is because she adheres to a humanist model of monstrosity that only understands monstrosity as a negative identity formation.

While paying careful attention here to the powerful counternarrative of a feminist pleasure in horror, I will also try to reestablish the terms of a reception of horror that manages to resituate the subtexts of race and class that the gendered narrative erases. It is important to first respond to the psychoanalytic master narrative of gendered fear by exposing the misogynist (and potentially homophobic) stakes of such a narrative, but it is equally important to realize that at any moment undesirable class others and undesirable racialized others may lurk behind the monster and/or the female victim. It is increasingly difficult to relay class and race back through the contemporary horror film because the emphasis upon the female victim as protagonist inevitably gives us a gendered lens through which to watch the action. The emergence within contemporary horror of a single female victim/protagonist, specifically a heroine who survives, replaces nineteenth-century Gothic fiction's series of almost indistinguishable female heroine/victims. This lone female figure forces horror to play in the key of gender in the contemporary horror film.

Race *as race* most often appears in horror films through minor characters who become body shields for the female victim and are infinitely expendable (see, for example, the function of people of color in *Aliens* or *Leviathan*). More often than not, however, race is wedded to the various demonized class identities and coded into the overall monstrosity of the monster. In this section I will focus upon the gender narrative in order to refute the dominant narratives of pleasure and displeasure validated by psychoanalysis, but I will also attempt to point to the places where disavowals of class and race appear in the psychoanalytic accounts of contemporary horror.

Carol Clover has recently challenged the conventional wisdom about the horror film which associated visual pleasure with a disturbing identification between a male gaze and monstrous violence against female bodies. Clover characterizes the horror film in terms of a "masochistic aesthetic" which locates the pleasure of watching horror for a male spectator not in "assaultive gazing" but in "the reactive or introjective position, figured as both painful and feminine."[16] Female paranoia may well be the counterpart to Clover's insistence upon the male's feminine masochism. If he is masochistic, she is paranoid and it is precisely the fear of being watched, the consciousness that we may be being watched, that saves the woman and allows her to look back. The women who are not worried about being watched within the horror film very often die; the alternative to paranoia in horror films very often is nothing more than a gullibility and a kind of stupid naivete. I am arguing, therefore, for a notion of productive fear which marks the female within Gothic as a subject who watches as well as a subject who is watched.

But the woman must also listen. As we saw in the case of paranoia, fear can also be produced from a sound: a click, a shutter (shudder?), "knocking." Productive fear, therefore, circulates through the power of the gaze but also through the power of directed listening. Within the structure of the horror film, furthermore, it is very often sound rather than sight that produces tension for the female viewer — soundtracks, for example, match and produce expected somatic responses to the images on the screen. The most famous horror soundtracks — the ones, for example, to *Psycho* and *Jaws* — are actually able to project stabbing and stalking through the medium of music. Very often the music transforms a spectator into a listener and then makes listening a part of the identifications between audience and victim or audience and slasher.

Alfred Hitchcock's classic horror film *The Birds* (1963) plays heavily with the auditory production of fear. I want to turn now to an analysis of *The Birds* in terms of female paranoia in order to suggest that very often horror films contain within their narrative strategies the seeds of feminist Gothic. *The Birds* has been heavily utilized in the past by psychoanalytic critics who are anxious to map out the sexual topography of the look and the cinematic structure of paranoia. Raymond Bellour, among others, has done detailed analyses of particular sequences in *The Birds* that link female sexuality to almost an essential victimhood.[17] Psychoanalytic readings of this film, I will argue, retrace Freud's steps through the case history of a female paranoiac. In other words, they use the connections between birds and women posited by the film only to suggest the complete subjugation of female sexuality within the narrative to an oedipalized male desire.

At least part of the power of horror within a contemporary context lies in the reception of horror as always very literally about the destruction of a woman. However, the horror narrative in its Gothic mode produces, as we have seen, multiple interpretations because of the mobilities of monstrosity. While Alfred Hitchcock's *The Birds* may not seem at first glance to be a Gothic text — there is, for example, no single monster — the birds in this film, visually and metaphorically, break monstrosity down into pieces. Furthermore, the birds represent quite literally the horror of nature *becoming* nature (birds becoming predatory) which in turn produces the almost supernatural events of the bird attacks. The

Gothic nature of this film lies in its insistence upon the multiplicity of readings for any set of weird phenomena, its seeming persecution of a single female victim, and its apparent alignment of female desire with excess and male desire with both conservatism and monstrosity. Obviously, there are other Hitchcock films which present themselves as more apparently Gothic (*Psycho*, most obviously) but this one codes both the punishment of femininity and the feminist potential of female aggression in both complex and readable ways.

In 1963 when *The Birds* was released, any number of social contexts might have given rise to the coding of fear as a fear of a mass of birds banding together in an artificial solidarity for the purpose of bombarding the exclusively white citizens of remote and elite communities like Bodega Bay. The rise of feminism, the civil rights movements, student activism, and the war in Vietnam surely all contributed to this particular manifestation of horror. *The Birds,* after all, refuses to locate fear or monstrosity in a singular and isolable body — very clearly, the horror that the birds represent is a horror predicated upon the unusual banding together of birds of a feather. It is interesting, then, to notice how little attention has been paid to sociopolitical accounts of the horror of the birds. In what follows I contribute to the existing debates about gender in *The Birds* but I also suggest that the overdetermination of the gender reading of the film has effectively blocked out the other readings.

Within *The Birds,* the birds themselves register their presence as sound; the accumulation of bird sounds comes to represent a menace to society. In the opening credits, a disharmonious symphony of bird song plays over the images of birds flitting like shadows across the credit titles; interestingly, the birds actually deform the titles as if their images and their voices can break down language into pieces or fragments of a much more complicated acoustic code. The noise of the birds immediately suggests danger although the actual physical threat they represent remains blurry and indistinct. The credits quickly give way to a shot of Melanie Daniels (Tippi Hedrun) walking across San Francisco's Union Square as a boy whistles at her. His whistle briefly replaces or fades into the cacophony of the bird soundtrack but is instantly erased again by an individual bird whistle which visibly scares Melanie. Many critics read this opening scene as the conflation of the birds and male sexuality; the boy's whistle becomes the sound of a desire which can turn instantly from desire to violence and become a slashing and penetrating attack. Also, Hitchcock's camera in this scene comes down from above, it conveys precisely a bird's-eye view and therefore situates the gaze of the auteur with the cry of the birds. However, as the film elaborates, there are equally powerful associations to be made between women and birds, particularly caged birds, and between women and a birdlike (harpy) form of violence.

One critic, Jacqueline Rose, has suggested the connections between female paranoia and feminist subversions of the cinematic apparatus using Hitchcock's *The Birds*. Rose's article is an intensely psychoanalytic reading of "paranoia and the film system" in which she argues for "the pertinence of the topographical concept of regression and that of paranoid projection for a metapsychology of film."[18] I understand her to mean that the paranoid projection provides an analogue to cinema and the gaze and that both transform fear and desire into visual space or topographies. In relation to the horror film, Rose claims that in its intent to "excite displeasure" (145), the horror film in particular resembles closely the mechanism of paranoia. Rose suggests that *The Birds* releases an excess of aggressivity within its paranoid projections even as it develops a diegetic and visual narrative around paranoia, narcissism, and psychosis. Rose writes:

> The birds themselves emanate from the inherent instability of the film's own system, overdetermined in this instance by a series of narrative relations which direct the energy of the film around the woman, while also using those positions to comment upon its own system of repression; by doing so it subsumes the excess of its own aggressivity into a meta-(psycho-)analysis defined as an act of knowledge. That the film is unable to cope with the aggressivity it releases is most clearly indicated by the resolution. (152)

For Rose the birds in Hitchcock's film represent precisely, we might say, psychic projectiles which Melanie creates and is attacked by. She is, Rose says, "both object and cause of the attack." Certainly the townspeople of Bodega Bay seem to agree. However, while Rose understands that the force of the violence of the birds allows for a potential release of female aggressivity that the film might not be able to contain, ultimately she reads female paranoia as a debilitating structure that must render the female mute and infantile before it resolves itself. Therefore, though Rose acknowledges that "the film is unable to cope with the aggressivity it releases," she ultimately claims that resolution comes "only at the expense of the woman" (153).

Another feminist critic also reads *The Birds* as a film which has the potential to unleash a particularly feminine form of aggressivity but that ultimately fails to capitalize on such potential. Susan Lurie, in "The Construction of the 'Castrated Woman' in Psychoanalysis and Cinema," makes the rather remarkable and useful claim that far from representing the truth of castration to the little boy, the woman reveals to the young male that "she is not castrated despite the fact that she has 'no penis,' and does inspire male fear for his castration."[19] The woman, within Lurie's rewriting of the scene of castration, represents a sexually "different" body that is not impaired by not possessing the penis. Lurie argues that the fiction of the "powerful castrated penis" is generated within psychoanalysis to establish the transcendence of castration over and above its irrelevance to the female body.

In her reading of *The Birds*, Lurie details the power of the female look and she notes the necessary disempowerment of the female in order to subjugate her under the fiction of castration. Lurie performs a close analysis of the Bodega Bay scene in which Melanie rides across the bay and back in a boat to deposit a gift of lovebirds at Mitch's house. This sequence has been structurally dissected by Raymond Bellour to analyze the dialectic of the look and to claim that Melanie Daniels is "equal and complicit in the look."[20] Lurie agrees with Bellour that Hitchcock is concerned with the vision of Melanie Daniels but, Lurie adds, only "to establish its severe limitations" (64). Lurie describes a "dark side of the look," one which attacks the looker from a place off camera and constructs a castrated woman. She understands the Bodega Bay boat ride to be a circumscription of Melanie's power of vision which culminates, of course, in the attack upon her of the gull which Mitch sees coming but which completely takes her by surprise. About the attack of the gull, Lurie states that "punishment for her desire, a desire the powerful look signifies, is the impairment of that look to the point of 'filling' it with the mark of that injury" (68).

While I agree with both Rose and Lurie that the birds in Hitchcock's film represent both the aggressivity of woman and her punishment, it seems to me that the punishment of the woman leads to yet another system of female paranoia, female aggression, and female violence. In order to expose this latter system and to appreciate its logic, however, we have to depart from the logic of psychoanalysis and its particular set of gender narratives. For both Rose and Lurie, the resolution to *The Birds* is a scene of total debilitation for the woman. Rose accepts Freud's universalizing interpretation of the female paranoiac as caught in the grips of a mother complex and she reads Melanie's decline at the end of the film, therefore, as a regressive identification with the mother which renders her infantile. Lurie, on the other hand, accepts the dominance of the myth of castration and reads Melanie's infantilization as a necessary step in making her safe for male desire. In both readings psychoanalytic accounts of female fear and desire prevail and the horror film must be understood as clearly operating on behalf of patriarchy. How can we disrupt such bleak but conclusive readings?

Certainly, after the attack upon her by the birds in the attic, Melanie Daniels has been reduced to a speechless hysteric who hallucinates imaginary birds and looks now without seeing. Throughout the film she has actively and aggressively pursued Mitch much to the disapproval of his mother and now finally she is completely under his power and his mother has become her mother as she becomes infantile. As the car finally drives away from the house, birds are thick upon the ground, gently cooing but gathering like a dark cloud in preparation for the next attack. The birds, grotesque in their awkward hopping and flapping, dominate the screen and fill it out completely as the car departs in defeat. The camera, both Lurie and Rose note, remains triumphantly perched among the conquering birds. A reading of this final scene in terms of Gothic feminist paranoia could easily break the terms of the psychoanalytic defeat of woman. We recall that, all along, birds—lovebirds, caged birds, wild birds, domestic birds—have been associated with women. Perhaps it is possible, therefore, to read the final scene as the triumph of a particular form of wild female power, a violent form of power represented by this flock or community of birds. The car, in this scene, holds the oedipalized family who must exit torn and tattered and leave the family home to its new occupants. The car literally represents what drives the family and its slow progression out of the frame signals the defeat, for now, of the oedipal family and its replacement with the birds—the chicks, the women—who watch as the car departs.

I will return to this scene of bird-watching and birds watching to claim for a feminist reading. First, we can see how insistently birds and women are matched up throughout the film. A paranoid Gothic reading of *The Birds* recognizes right away that femininity in this horror film resides in the birds themselves as much as in the female characters. Femininity here characterizes both monster and victim and the film places femininity always alongside transgression. But again, the transpositions

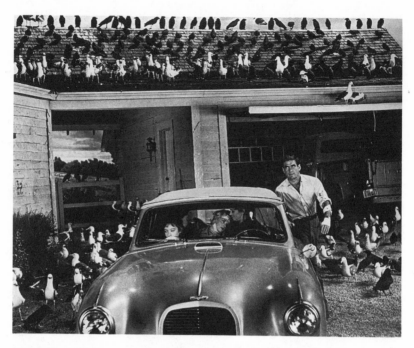

One of the last shots from Alfred Hitchcock's *The Birds*. The oedipal family drives off, leaving the birds victorious.

between the gender of the victim and the gender of horror leave unasked all kinds of questions about other registers of fear. The birds also present menace through the highly uncharacteristic activity of their massing together against a mutual enemy. It is easy to read into this image a proletarian image of the masses, the disenfranchised in class and race terms, rising up (literally) against their masters and swarming through towns and cities with revolutionary zeal. Once again, psychoanalytic accounts of the power of horror cannot even approach such a reading; a feminist counternarrative about *The Birds* upsets the neatness of the psychoanalytic frame and sets the stage for a whole host of other readings.

Woman, in *The Birds*, is always on the wrong side of the law, either as victim or as criminal. In Freud's essay on female paranoia, we recall, a lawyer turns the female paranoiac over to Freud when he "recognizes the pathological stamp of this accusation." Appeals to the law by women are most often read as pathological or simply untenable. A film like *The Birds* actually exposes the ways in which the law does not work for women as long as men symbolically represent the law and its limits. At the end of the first meeting in the pet shop between Mitch and Melanie, we find out that Melanie is a criminal whom Mitch has encountered in court because she broke a "plate glass window" during a practical joke. Of course, birds repeatedly break windows during the film. They attack Melanie through a phone booth, they smash a young girl's glasses, and they punch out old man Fawcett's eyes and his truck windows. The window is a screen that should protect but be invisible; only when it breaks does it become visible and penetrable, like the movie screen through which horror threatens to break. The birds also here penetrate the place of vision, the look, in order to blind and blinker certain forms of vision.

Lydia, Mitch's mother, similarly establishes herself as outside of the law, telling Mitch, "never mind the law." Maternal power seems at least temporarily to exist in a realm above the law. Mitch, on the other hand, is bound by the law; he is a lawyer and therefore limited like the police to a supervisory role. He is always a spectator, rarely an object or subject; he is subsumed, as Lydia tells him, by the portrait of his father who represents the real law in the house, the law of oedipal desire. The oedipal family—made up of Lydia, Mitch, Melanie, Kathy, and Annie—becomes the real target for the birds who break into the house and replace the family unit with the mass or tribe that their flock represents. Annie is the first of the family to go and she is identified all along as the outsider to the law of the family but also as what the family insistently rejects. Annie does not reject the family, it rejects her and identifies her as surplus. The film names Melanie as her successor—she is Mel-anie, another version of Annie but one who is willing to succumb to the law of oedipal desire.

Within all of the main attack scenes in the film, the birds' aggressiveness seems to be inspired by the attempts of characters to cohere as family within a romantic narrative. Of course, as we have already noted, the film underscores the connection between romance or desire and the birds' aggression in the opening scenes of the film when the boy's whistle at Melanie is followed by the bird's whistle. The boy's whistle may be a call of desire but the bird's whistle is definitely a warning. Following Annie's and Melanie's discussion of Mitch and his mother, a bird hurls itself at Annie's front door as if to portend the violence that the family narrative produces. The two women stand at the door in the moonlight and look down upon the bird; this is a threshold moment in the film, a moment when one potential narrative, a narrative about desires between women, is subsumed by another narrative, a heterosexual romance. The dead bird at the doorstep suggests the violence that is required in order for the family romance narrative to assert itself.

.This scene is preceded by an earlier moment of bird aggression, the one Lurie reads so closely, the scene in the bay. Melanie's ride back across Bodega Bay represents her at her most powerful. She has crept like a criminal into Mitch's house and planted the symbolic seeds of destruction, the lovebirds, which will soon be replaced by the hate birds that similarly slip unnoticed into the familial mansion. Melanie drives the boat confidently and with authority while Mitch watches her from the dock. The camera performs shot / reverse shots in order to share the look between Mitch and Melanie. As Melanie drives she cocks her head and looks almost quizzically towards shore resembling nothing so much as a bird. Certainly, when the bird pecks at her, swooping down upon her from off camera, Melanie's triumph is turned to humiliation. The trickle of blood left by the bird's beak suggests a deflowering of sorts and it is here that the decline of Melanie's power begins.

The birds attack first when romance starts up between Mitch and Melanie; once again, in the attack, the birds seem almost to have pinpointed the oedipalized scene of romance and then swooped down upon it. The next day at the children's party, the birds attack again during a game of blindman's bluff. The birds attack women and children and they always attack when no one is looking. Like the famous scene where the birds slowly accumulate behind Melanie on a children's climbing frame in the schoolyard, the birds are always precisely working behind the scene, growing in numbers and preparing to attack scenes of domesticity in order to replace them with a wild, swarming, flapping, noisy femininity. And the domestic tranquility that the birds destroy stands in for other forms of quiet oppression like white racism and a corrupt class system.

I want to look at one final scene in the film to establish conclusively the link that *The Birds* insists upon and then disrupts between women and birds and women and paranoia. Following another attack on school children, Melanie ends up in the town cafe where a conversation takes place between Mrs. Bundy, an ornithologist, and the cook in the cafe who claims that the birds portend the end of the world. The gender configurations in this scene are quite interesting in that the male is associated with religion and cooking and the female with science. A spontaneous town meeting springs up around the conversation between Bundy and the cook and people put forth their various theories of the birds. Throughout, Mrs. Bundy veers between the voice of reason and a kind of Cassandra voice of doom. On the one hand, she claims that birds are not aggressive, it is man who is aggressive. Furthermore, she argues, birds of different species don't flock together. On the other hand, she warns, if the birds were aggressive and if they did flock together, then "we wouldn't have a chance."

The birds attack again, bombing down upon the townspeople outside, trapping Melanie in a glass phone booth and effectively cutting off all means of communication with the outside world. (The birds are often seen gathering on phone wires as if they begin their work like an efficient military expedition by cutting off the lines to the outside world.) Melanie runs back into the cafe and is greeted by the most extraordinary scene in the film. The cafe is empty except for a group of huddled casualties, all women and children, lining the corridor. The wounded stare at Melanie with accusatory expressions and the camera slowly pans their faces. Finally someone screams at Melanie, lashing out at her and accusing her of bringing the birds to Bodega Bay. This scene remarkably plays with the paranoid conspiracy theories that had been tossed around the cafe and reduces them to one theory which demands a scapegoat. Melanie is now responsible for the birds, she represents the birds and their aggressivity and they represent her. From now on, as she draws ever closer to Mitch and as the family home becomes her cage and prison, the birds will batter and bomb the house until it gives way and relinquishes the domestic female.

The birds, in this film, very literally represent the power that could potentially be released by the spectacle of different species of women (or different classes or races) flocking together. If they did that, Mrs. Bundy warns, "we wouldn't have a chance." The "we" in this sentence obviously stands for "human" but the distinction between human and bird insistently breaks down through the film as birds become aggressive and humans become defensive. The narrative of romance, humanism, and family values that underwrites both the story of Mitch, Melanie, and Lydia and also the story of the people of Bodega Bay (closing ranks against outsiders) is under severe attack here from the narrative of a unified and intentional attack from above by harpies whose intent seems clearly to break down the structures of heterosexual desire and replace them with a female homosociality.

To return one final time to Freud's case history of paranoia in a woman, Freud claims to have found the homosexual component to the paranoid fantasy when he uncovers a mother complex in his young patient. The paranoid fantasy now becomes a defense against the supposedly insupportable desire of a woman for another woman. Apart from the fact that Freud here subsumes female fear under the model of male fear and refuses to validate the woman's quite reasonable anxiety about being watched, what is at stake in the discovery of the mother complex is a homophobic construction of lesbian desire as untenable and even pathological. *The Birds* plays with the notion of a mother complex by creating a mother-daughter bond between Lydia and Melanie. In the human sphere of action in the film, aggressive femininity and paranoid femininity are precisely punished as Melanie loses her voice, her love object (Mitch), and possibly her sanity. But the birds — the figments of her paranoid imagination that seem to invisibly attack her at the end of the film — the birds represent the alternative to Freud's (and possibly Hitchcock's) reading of female paranoia. The birds, by the film's resolution, become the ones that watch, the ones that stalk, the ones that occupy Bodega Bay. In contrast to Melanie — the lovebird — who now lies mute, the wild birds are out of the gilded cage and have entered a new frame of desire.

Conclusion

Throughout this chapter I have tried to argue that paranoia, like Gothic, is never wholly reactionary nor wholly liberatory. Paranoia, furthermore, has the peculiar property of tending to produce the reality it fears. In Freud's analyses of two cases of paranoia, one in a man and one in a woman, he ratifies a particular psychoanalytic narrative about fear and desire by locating pathological fear in a horror of homosexual desire and an equally horrific prospect of evolving femininity. Furthermore, Freud refuses to acknowledge the specificities of the female case of paranoia, indeed the local, political, and cultural specificities of female fear in patriarchy, and he simply models the female case of paranoia upon the male case. I have chosen here to read with, rather than against, the female paranoiac in order to demonstrate that fear can be productive and that horror narratives are not always and everywhere complicit with misogyny. Monstrosity is often coded female or else transformed by the end of the film or narrative into a pathological form of femininity.

The triumph of psychoanalytic narratives of human fear and desire is evident in the oppositions within contemporary horror between the monstrous and the female. No matter what the shape or form of monstrosity, it is a female victim who runs screaming into the void. For this reason the class and race components to the generativity of the monster become hidden by the gender and sexuality of the monster. The female victim seems to demand a male or masculine predator. This is not to say that race and class have dropped out of the picture. As we saw in relation to a counterreading of *The Birds,* the horror of the birds is as easily associated by the viewer with the supposed horror of the masses coming together to assault the cozy existence of the middle classes. It is equally plausible to read the aggressive birds as aggrieved people of color, bonding together in their joint enterprise against white homeowners. Certainly such codes are in place in *The Birds* and certainly they register with viewers on some level. However, the visual and narrative emphases upon the female victim as female (as opposed to say the representative of Englishness or whiteness or Americanness or middle-class humanity) draws the spectator to gendered and sexualized frames of reference for everything else that follows.

In the next chapter we will see what happens if we deploy not simply feminist but queer readings of what looks like gender horror in order to establish the possibility of a powerful female monstrosity and a debilitating male fear.

Bodies That Splatter:

Queers and Chain Saws

Show me what I fear so I don't fear it no more.
—*Dennis Hopper,* THE TEXAS CHAINSAW MASSACRE 2

Bodies that Splatter

The horror film has typically been theorized as a misogynist genre that provides a showcase for masculine aggression and provokes a sexual response to the spectacle of female mutilation. Such a view of horror film seems borne out by audience surveys which suggest that young males make up the primary group that watches horror films. This chapter pressures the formulation of horror as masculine pleasure and, following on from my last chapter on the productive nature of female or feminist paranoia, we will see if, when, and how the horror film can be recuperated for feminine, feminist, and queer forms of pleasure. Furthermore, in keeping with the themes of this book, I want to examine the Gothic technologies of subject production as they operate through the apparatus of the contemporary horror film. In a film like *The Texas Chainsaw Massacre 2* (1986), gender, race, class, and sexuality are thoroughly scrambled as categories and what emerges are queer identity formations literally sutured together from the scraps of flesh that survive the chain saw.

The category "horror film" at this point covers a vast range of cinema; included in this genre are slasher/splatter films (e.g. *Halloween, Friday the 13th, A Nightmare on Elm Street, The Texas Chainsaw Massacre*), Gothic psychothrillers (*Psycho, The Birds, The Silence of the Lambs*), sci-fi horror (*Alien*), rape revenge (*The Accused, Ms. 45*), supernatural horror (*The Exorcist*). In this chapter I pay careful attention to a few examples of the slasher/splatter film as precisely the location of the dismantling and reconstruction of bodily identities and also of spectatorial positions, gazes, and desires. John McCarty, in *Splatter Movies*, defines splatter films as "offshoots of the horror film genre" which "aim not to scare their audiences, nor to drive them to the edge of their seats in suspense, but to mortify them with explicit gore." He sums up: "In splatter movies, mutilation is the message."[1] In keeping with the transitions that I have been charting from the horror associated with landscapes and houses in the eighteenth-century Gothic Romance to the horror of Gothic monstrous bodies in the nineteenth century, the splatter film occupies a key place in terms of the preoccupation in the twentieth century with not simply the external monstrosities of the body but the increasingly voyeuristic quest to show what lies below the skin.

One recent book on horror has radically altered the conditions of horror film theory. *Men, Women and Chain Saws* by Carol Clover proposes that the radical potential of the horror film lies in the identification it forces between the male viewer and the female victim (a masochistic viewer position). Clover writes: "Cinefantastic horror, in short, succeeds in incorporating its spectators as 'feminine' and then violating that body—which recoils, shudders, cries out collectively—in ways otherwise imaginable for males only in nightmare."[2] Clover is less clear about the potential identification that horror allows between the female viewer and the male or female aggressor. She also has a tendency to restabilize gendered positions in relation to horror. The queer tendency of horror film, in my opinion, lies in its ability to reconfigure gender not simply through inversion but by literally creating new categories. For example, the relations between femininity and chain saws in *The Texas Chainsaw Massacre 2* significantly alter the terrain and bodily space of the "girl" in these films. Similarly, the relations between men and a splattered masculinity significantly affects the meanings of maleness.

Obviously, my title for this chapter, "Bodies That Splatter," recalls Judith Butler's book *Bodies That Matter* and poses the problem of which bodies matter in terms of the question of which bodies splatter. *Bodies That Matter* is on some levels a continuation of Butler's earlier project *Gender Trouble*. In *Bodies That Matter*, she takes up again the ways in which genders are produced and performed through bodies and subjectivities as repetitions or citations of a phantasmatic ideal of gender identity. As an example of the ways in which we manufacture gender, Butler gives the following: "Consider the medical interpellation which . . .

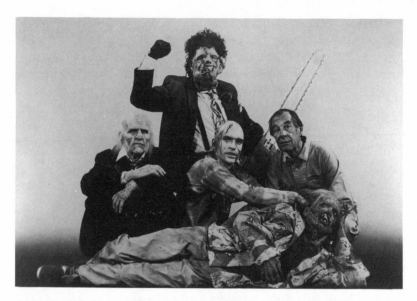

Publicity still from *The Texas Chainsaw Massacre, Part 2.*

shifts an infant from an 'it' to a 'she' or a 'he,' and in that naming, the girl is 'girled,' brought into the domain of language and kinship through the interpellation of gender."[3] The idea that females are "girled" produces gender as a material effect of naming and presents the problem of whether and how one might intervene in the process of girling in order to disrupt the even flow of gendering. Obviously, girling is interrupted repeatedly, and inevitably in fact, and this is what makes gender identity into a rough shape rather than a smooth surface of social construction. It is in the failures of gendering, girling and boying, that gender construction becomes visible.

Linking gender construction to the category of humanness, Butler writes:

[T]he construction of gender operates through exclusionary means, such that the human is not only produced over and against the inhuman, but through a set of foreclosures, radical erasures, that are, strictly speaking, refused the possibility of cultural articulation. Hence, it is not enough to claim that human subjects are constructed, for the construction of the human is a differential operation that produces the more and less "human," the inhuman, the humanly unthinkable. (8)

Of course, as Butler implies, it is not only improper gender that becomes allied with inhumanity. The construction of race and class also "operate through exclusionary means." However, gender bears a certain proximity to the human within modern contexts because, as Michel Foucault's work has amply shown, the history of sexuality culminates in the production of individuated subjects who experience sexuality and gender as part of their core identity.

Gender construction and its failures in particular open out onto the category of the human which appears at the limits of proper gender as the "inhuman," or the "less than human." In other words, improperly or inadequately gendered bodies represent the limits of the human and they present a monstrous arrangement of skin, flesh, social mores, pleasures, dangers, and wounds. The bodies that splatter in horror films are interestingly enough properly gendered "human" bodies, female bodies, in fact, with all the conventional markings of their femininity. Female bodies that do not splatter, then, are often sutured bodies, bodies that are in some way distanced from the gender constructions that would otherwise sentence them to messy and certain death. Carol Clover has named the improperly gendered, de-girled being as the "final girl."

The final girl is, according to Clover, the survivor; "the one who encounters the mutilated bodies of her friends and perceives the full extent of the preceding horror and of her own peril; who is chased, cornered, wounded; whom we see scream, stagger, fall, rise, and scream again" (35). As the character who lives to tell the tale of horror, the final girl, Clover argues, must be accessible as a point of identification to male viewers. For this reason the final girl's gender is ambiguous. "The final girl is boyish," (40) says Clover and she adds, "what filmmakers seem to know better than film critics is that gender is less a wall than a permeable membrane" (46). Gender, we might add, drawing from earlier formulations of identity in this project, is often a very specific "permeable membrane"—the skin. Someone's skin, their hide (Hyde), precisely forms the surface through which inner identities emerge and upon which external readings of identity leave their impression. The Texas Chainsaw Massacre 2, in fact, provides its viewers with a virtual skinfest and constantly focuses upon skin and the shredding, ripping, or tearing of skin as a spectacle of identity performance and its breakdown.

The spectacle of skin in Dr. Jekyll and Mr. Hyde, as we saw, simultaneously signified the hiding of sex and race; in The Texas Chainsaw Massacre 2, the dominance of the narrative action by the female protagonist makes race virtually unreadable. However, as Clover again has pointed out, in its generic affinities to the western, the horror film does have a way of coding monstrosity in ethnic terms as white trash, rednecks, or redskins. Clover writes: "If 'redneck' once denoted a real and particular group, it has achieved the status of a kind of universal blame figure, the 'someone else' held responsible for all manner of American social ills. The great success of the redneck in that capacity suggests that anxieties no longer expressible in ethnic or racial terms have become projected onto a safe target" (135). This is an extremely important account of what happens to the whole category of racial monstrosity in American horror film. As I noted in chapter 1, the expression of racial fear in a contemporary context has become inseparable from racism. This does not mean, however, that racial coding disappears from the horror film; rather it becomes, as I have already suggested and as Clover eloquently elaborates, part of the class or regional makeup of the monster. In *The Texas Chainsaw Massacre 2,* the Sawyer family certainly plays the part of the rednecks living beyond the purview of urban civilization and they also bear the trappings of cinematic "redskins" with their skins, hides, and fetish feather objects.

The Texas Chainsaw Massacre 2 signifies, within my project, as a paradigmatic example of skin horror. While the postmodern horror film does not tend to produce what we have been calling, with Moretti, "totalizing" monsters, the Sawyer family is perhaps as close as we get. As we will see in *The Silence of the Lambs,* monstrosity finally fades out of the picture when the monstrous becomes coextensive with the normal and indeed the dominant. Buffalo Bill and Hannibal Lecter represent an inverted couple who embody monstrosity as an effect of dominant rather than subversive notions of taste, fashion, domesticity, and identity. In *The Texas Chainsaw Massacre 2,* Tobe Hooper lingers upon skin and its shredding with a sado-pornographic eye for detail and a finely tuned sense of the metonymic uses and abuses of skin. Human interaction, in this Gothic orgy, is literalized as skin trade, and shedding and wearing, flaying and tanning, ripping and sewing become the practices, the specifically sexual practices, of a subterranean group of skin jobs.

Furthermore, *The Texas Chainsaw Massacre 2* confronts the viewer with possibly the most virile, certainly the most heroic, and definitely the most triumphant final girl in splatter film. Stretch is a screamer alright, but her screaming is a Diamanda Galas-like soundtrack to her own blood opera. If the empowerment of women in *The Birds,* as we saw in the last chapter, occurs subtly and stealthily through the image of the gathering of the masses, female power in *The Texas Chainsaw Massacre 2* is channeled through the perfect antidote to the hapless, aristocratic, lethargic Gothic heroine—a white trash bitch with a chain saw. Stretch not only saves the day in this film, she saves herself and learns how to be a monster. In *The Texas Chainsaw Massacre 2,* then, by contrast to the action in the previous film, *The Texas Chainsaw Massacre,* as we shall see, we witness the becoming-monstrous of a woman which does not automatically mean that she must compromise herself, sacrifice her voice, or give up her hard-won gains to a man. The chain saw massacre in *The Texas Chainsaw Massacre 2,* as opposed to the gorefest at the female's expense in *The Texas Chainsaw Massacre,* is a massacre of Stretch's making.

I intend to read Stretch as a Gothic heroine who transforms the function of woman within the Gothic text to, finally, a function that is part of the technology of monsters and that transforms the category of monster itself into an orgiastic celebration of the queer and the dangerous. Usually within Gothic technologies of monstrosity, as we have seen, the monster works as a kind of trash heap for the discarded scraps of abject humanity. Monster-making, I have argued throughout, is a suspect activity because it relies upon and shores up conventional humanist binaries. The technology of monsters when channeled through a dangerous woman with a chain saw becomes a powerful and queer strategy for enabling and activating monstrosity as opposed to stamping it out.

Gender works quite differently through Stretch than through other final girls. While Clover's formulation of the final girl and her function as a channel for the male gaze is compelling, there is a way in which she remains caught in a gender lock. The world of female victims and male monsters remains intact in Clover's reading and only lines of identification or gazes shift focus. What I want to argue is that the final girl, particularly as embodied by Stretch, represents not boyishness or girlishness but monstrous gender, a gender that splatters, rips at the seams, and then is sutured together again as something much messier than male or female. Linda Williams has argued exactly this in "When the Woman Looks" and she claims that while "the male look expresses conventional fear at that which differs from itself," the female look "shares the male's fear of the monster's freakishness, but also recognizes the sense in which this freakishness is similar to her own difference."[4] Williams goes on to suggest that the woman's look and her monstrosity have subversive potential but are too often soundly punished within the horror film. Perhaps what is lacking from Williams's analysis is a sense that the woman's monstrosity and her relation to violence in the horror film changes profoundly the form of her gender itself. Gender is monstrous in the horror film and it exceeds even the category of human. The genders that emerge triumphant at the gory conclusion of a splatter film are literally posthuman, they punish the limits of the human body and they mark identities as always stitched, sutured, bloody at the seams, and completely beyond the limits and the reaches of an impotent humanism.

If, traditionally, splatter films have not been watched by women and girls because female bodies were precisely the ones most likely to splatter, then a space of viewership has to be reopened in order to reconstitute potential gazes. As we have seen throughout this study, Gothic contains great potential for a kind of interactive dynamic between text and viewers. The suppleness of monstrosity allows for numerous interventions in the business of interpretations. It is precisely on account of the interactive potential of the horror text that female viewership and readership becomes essential to the production of meaning. In her study of spectatorship, Clover carried out impromptu and casual surveys of her local video store in order to acquire information about who watched what within the genre of the horror film. Such a survey, of course, is completely unreliable since, as she fully acknowledges, men could be renting videos for women at home, boys might be renting them for their sisters, girlfriends, or mothers. It is, however, probable that, as Linda Williams phrases it, "whenever the movie screen holds a particularly effective image of terror, little boys and grown men make it a point of honor to look, while little girls and grown women cover their eyes or hide behind the shoulders of their dates" (88). Ignoring, for a moment, the heterosexist presumption of this formulation (grown women are with male dates at the movies), it is worth asking with Williams what happens "when the woman looks." In order to begin to answer this question, we must produce reevaluations of the horror film in terms of potential feminist or woman-positive readings which make horror available to the female viewer. Furthermore, we might examine Williams's heterosexist faux pas long enough to note that homophobia tends to run alongside misogyny within the horror film and both are often expressed as a violence against gender instability. In what follows I will try to explain the particular potential of the queer or antihomophobic look while also attending to what happens when the woman looks.

Another reason that it is often difficult for a horrorphobic female or viewer to watch a splatter film is because, as we have noted, horror works hard at dismantling the stable relations between representation and reality. And feminists in particular have not always been very attuned to the nuances that structure the relationship between representation and reality. The pornography debates of the 1980s repeatedly staged the hypothesis that representations of the violation of female bodies produce the actual rape and battery of women.[5] Similarly, feminist responses to the horror film have tended to question whether representations of violence against women would produce actual violence.

Obviously, the relationship between representation and reality is always vexed and unclear and certainly any feminist consideration of horror must take this into consideration. But in fact, it is very useful to begin by acknowledging that there is a difference between violence and its representation and that the task of interpretation is not to pinpoint what this difference is but rather to ask how the confusion between representation and reality works to produce fear and horror. Horror film very often situates itself upon the slippage between representations and their material effects.

Wes Craven's *A Nightmare on Elm Street* (1984) not only exemplifies the ways in which horror film exploits the tension between representation and reality, it actually makes this tension into its primary theme. The narrative in *Nightmare* is motored by the notion that dream life is contaminated by real horror and that real horror might be contaminated by dreams. The girl in this film who negotiates the difference between dreaming and waking most successfully will live to scream/dream again. In *Nightmare* a group of teenagers are all haunted in their dreams by the figure of Freddy Krueger, a child murderer who had been killed by a mob of parents. One by one the teenagers are visited and brutalized by the man with knives for fingers until only Nancy and her boyfriend, played by Johnny Depp, remain. (Depp plays a beefcake boyfriend here but in his next dramatic role he appears as a kind of castrated Freddy Krueger, the wimpy Edward Scissorhands.) Nancy wages war on Freddy by trying to sort out the tangled relation between dreamscape, real time, and actual bodily mutilation.

This film, in fact, radically advocates for an active and aggressive spectatorship which does, as Clover might argue, feminize the audience but also empowers them. Nancy is a participant/spectator who repeatedly calls attention to herself as spectator—"it's only a dream"—and pulls herself out of dream states by physically hurting herself. In other words, she attempts always to remain embodied, to be aware of what it means to have a body, and to understand how that body can be hurt by unconscious drifting. This film suggests that it is dangerous to leave your body in the theater, watching must be an alert and self-conscious process as opposed to the conventional notions of spectatorship as a kind of escape into passive inertia. It is when you cease to watch yourself watching that you become the victim.

In the final encounter between Nancy and Krueger, however, Nancy, of course, articulates an even more powerful model of spectatorship, one which can alter what will happen by trapping the monster, pulling him into reality, and then "turning one's back on him" in order to draw energy away. Several techniques of spectatorship are at work here. First, horror depends upon energy directed at the screen, not just energy directed at the viewer — you are only scared if you want to be. Second, readings of monsters *can* disable them. Nancy actually sets out to interpret her dream and thus to disarm it. While her mother calls upon the dubious authority of a sleep disorder clinic to unravel the problem of dreaming, Nancy recognizes that the clinic cannot produce a solution because their theory of the relation between the body and the imagination is limited by the medical technology that sees bodies as highly manipulable and easily read. You need a more complicated theory of dreams and pleasure and bodies in order to counter Freddy Krueger. Nancy comes up with one — he is *her* dream and *her* nightmare and if she is able to collapse the real and the imagined long enough to banish him, then she will win.

Keeping the appropriate distance between representations and reality is one way for a girl to survive Gothic horror and slasher films but there are others. In *The Texas Chainsaw Massacre 2*, femininity or girlness itself is recycled and transformed into new and different gender regimes. As we will see, relations between sex and gender, reality and representation in this film are not simply inverted, they are altogether reconstructed.

Facing Off: The Texas Chainsaw Massacre 2

The Texas Chainsaw Massacre 2 takes up from *The Texas Chainsaw Massacre,* the story of a cannibalistic Texas family, the Sawyers (sewers? saw-ers?), who recycle human flesh into chili. The townspeople consume the famous Sawyer chili and thereby become implicated in a kind of large-scale cannibalism, a cannibalism that actually defines the local modes of production and consumption. Furthermore, as horror critic Robin Wood points out, the cannibalism exemplifies the practices associated with the capitalist family. "The family, after all," he writes, "only carries to its logical conclusion the basic (though unstated) tenet of capitalism, that people have the right to live off other people."[6] The cycle of chain saw massacres carried out by Leatherface and his bizarre brother Chop Top to provide meat for the chili comes to a halt when Lefty, played by Dennis Hopper, comes to town seeking vengeance on the Sawyers for their earlier murder of his nephew and niece. Lefty is joined in battle against the Sawyers by a local female DJ called Stretch. The second half of the film involves a series of bloody encounters between Stretch and the Sawyers and Lefty and the Sawyers in the Sawyer den — a labyrinthine underground structure that houses their culinary exploits and resembles nothing so much as an intestinal cavern.

This film stages a number of interesting "face offs" that pit strange forces against each other; for example, part of the horror of the chain saw attacks emanates from the loud and insistent growling of the live tool itself. The buzzing of the chain saw, however, is countered by Stretch's own noisemaking — she is a DJ who works in a soundproof booth and represents the power of noise rather than the noise of power. Her radio station, interestingly enough, sits atop a gun shop as if to emphasize the ballistic power of, not the gaze, but the sound wave. To take this opposition further, Stretch has put herself in the line of fire because she accidentally records a chain saw massacre when two college boys are murdered on the air. They call in to give requests and harass Stretch when they are attacked by the Sawyers. Stretch tapes the gruesome sounds of the massacre and then plays the tape on the air to try to find witnesses to the murder. Here the recycling of human flesh that characterizes the Sawyer family faces off against the recycling of sound that defines Stretch's job. Stretch literally plays back to the Sawyers the sounds of their own violence. It is no surprise, then, that she ultimately finishes the family off by playing them their own tune — she picks up the chain saw and performs her own cover version of the chain saw song.

Chainsaw 2 very specifically faces off against *Chainsaw*. *Chainsaw*, as Clover points out, almost belongs to a different genre of horror film because the female victim has to be rescued by male intervention and is not exactly representative of the final girls who follow her. Also, *Chain-*

saw simply looks different from *Chainsaw 2*. It presents itself as realistic docudrama while *Chainsaw 2* is pure fantasy, lurid and graphic, and often it comes close to animation with its heavy reliance on special effects. *Chainsaw* was released in 1974 and it has come to occupy a kind of cult position within the history of horror. Christopher Sharrett, in "The Idea of Apocalypse in *The Texas Chainsaw Massacre*," argues that the film has been incorrectly categorized as a "slasher" film and he predictably goes on to argue for the film as somehow larger than its low genre classification. He says it "represents a crucial moment in the history of the horror genre, when the form develops a specific relationship to the historical and cultural trend discussed and to a distinct period of discontent in American society."[7] Of course, as I have been saying throughout this project, the horror genre always bears a "specific relationship" to cultural and political trends and it is unconvincing, therefore, if not anticlimactic, to argue for *The Texas Chainsaw Massacre* as the "crucial moment" when horror finally reflects upon political contexts. Also, it is interesting that in order to make a claim for the importance of this film within the history of horror, Sharrett has to simultaneously argue that it goes beyond the generic field. Still, the usefulness of Sharrett's article lies in his willingness to situate the film in relation to a whole host of historically specific cultural anxieties about societal decline, about Watergate, and about cannibalism and capitalism.

Chainsaw is actually an intensely artsy film despite its low-budget production values. Articles about the making of the film stress the precision and care that went into its production.[8] An interview by John Mc-Carty with one of the actors in *Chainsaw* reveals that Hooper rose to the challenge of working with a tiny budget ($140,000) and in primitive conditions. The actor explains the eventual phenomenal success of the film as a result of the craft and artistic will of Hooper. This film was strangely beautiful, well acted, and more importantly, it avoided the moral framework of most horror films. "*Chainsaw* was different," explains the actor, "it didn't have good and bad people in it. It just had stranger and stranger."[9]

Of course, scarcely a drop of blood is spilt on screen in *Chainsaw*. Mostly uncanny effects arise through camera angles and the creation of odd cramped screen space rather than through overt images of chain saw mutilation. Furthermore, the film's introduction with its documentary style voice-over narration warns the viewer of the real-life story about to be presented and effectively erases the comfortable space between fantasy and reality for the spectator. Also, this film, like *Psycho* and *The Silence of the Lambs,* was loosely based upon the real-life exploits of serial killer Ed Gein, the Wisconsin farmer who skinned his victims and made clothes and household objects out of their hides. *The Texas Chainsaw Massacre 2,* by contrast, makes no truth claims and seems to revel in its special effects.

The relationship between these two films, actually, is not unlike the relation of *Frankenstein* to *Dracula* in terms of the various strategies and methods for generating horror. While the earlier film creates atmospheric tension and lingers on the proximity between the sublime and the terrible, the later *Chainsaw* film goes straight for the throat and denies the viewer nothing in terms of splatter viewing. Reviews of *Chainsaw 2* seem to find that the film realizes the true gore potential of *Chainsaw.* If *Chainsaw* was artsy because it showed restraint, *Chainsaw 2* is artless because it revels in the visual details of a slaughter. In *Chainsaw* the spectacle of the chain saw, the presence of Leatherface, and the remnants of other victims all produced a creepy effect without ever having to show chain saw against flesh. In *Chainsaw 2* Hooper acts as if he has prepped his audience and is now ready to slice and dice. *Chainsaw 2* was made on a much bigger budget but it has never received the same kind of critical attention as its predecessor.[10]

The Sawyer house in *Chainsaw* is an aboveground structure as opposed to the slime pit in *Chainsaw 2* and while, in *Chainsaw 2,* human remains are strewn around the basement as bloody trophies that produce a visceral response in the viewer, in *Chainsaw* the house is actually beautifully decorated with bones and skulls, skin and spare body parts that seem to call for aesthetic appraisal. What *Chainsaw 2* vivifies, *Chainsaw* aestheticizes. While cannibalism in *Chainsaw 2* is a parodic enactment of capitalist enterprise, in *Chainsaw* it is a reaction to the ravages of capitalism. The Sawyer family members in the earlier narrative are unemployed slaughterhouse managers and their reaction to being out of work is to "use everything" that comes their way and transform the banal into the grotesquely beautiful.

The Sawyer mansion in *Chainsaw* is a surreal space where the machinic and the slimy meet and conjoin. In the garden mechanical objects hang on trees, in the house furnishings are mechanized body parts. In both films the true nature of the Sawyer enterprise is revealed when a tooth is discovered on the premises (*Chainsaw*) or in the chili (*Chainsaw 2*). The tooth represents the last fragment of the presence of a human body. It precisely represents identity (including the pun "dent"-ure within i-dent-ity) and the loss of anything like human identity. It is the smallest fragment of the body and its isolation suggests the decimation of the rest of the body.

Finally, from *Chainsaw* to *Chainsaw 2* a very noticeable shift takes place precisely in the relation of surface and depth. In *Chainsaw* the soon-to-be-murdered teenagers approach the Sawyer mansion one by one, and one by one they peer into the house through a screen door. The camera plays insistently with the shot/reverse shot to emphasize both the presence of something/someone within the house and also the function of the door as "screen" and as a thin dividing line between inside and outside, nature and technology, innocence and violence. Once the teenagers pass through the screen door, they enter a world that resembles nothing so much as the backside of a mirror. Values and bodies are inverted and turned inside out as the Sawyer enterprise consumes them whole. In *Chainsaw 2* the relation between surface and depth is exemplified by the subterranean structure of the Sawyer den — it literally tunnels below the surface of the city and it specifically sits below an abandoned amusement park. The circuslike horror of the rotting sideshows opens up to the bleeding walls of the Sawyer abyss. But while space in this film seems to be organized according to a rather conventional sense of surface and depth, identity is not. *Chainsaw 2* fixates upon identity as surface, as skin. While *Chainsaw* seems interested in giving psychological explanations for horror and gruesome behavior, *Chainsaw 2* cannot validate the psychological reading.

Facing off in the *Chainsaw* films balances opposition and similarity with a difference alongside each other and then embodies this definition within one character — Leatherface. Leatherface is perhaps the most interesting member of the Sawyer family. He looks like a walking accident because of his mutilated face and his clumsy and sexual handling of his chain saw. Leatherface's role is somewhat limited in *Chainsaw* and his battle with the screaming girl (Marilyn Burns) is repetitive and not particularly distinctive. In *Chainsaw 2* the relationship between these two characters focuses the change in positionality of victimhood, power, monstrosity, violence, and desire within Gothic splatter films.

In a series of showdowns (face offs) in *Chainsaw 2* between Leatherface and Stretch, attack turns into romance as they circle each other in a crazy dance of flesh and desire. In the first encounter, Leatherface points his chain saw at Stretch's crotch in a blatantly sexual mode. When he appears to reach a frenzy of orgasm precisely by challenging Stretch but not by cutting her, he develops a brutal romantic attachment to her. For the rest of the film, Stretch manages to play with his desire in order to escape his blade.

Leatherface is the "chef" at the Sawyer den. His job is to prep the human flesh and turn it into meat. This means skinning it and taking out the organs. In one paradigmatic scene, Stretch peers over a trash can filled with human debris to watch Leatherface's culinary exploits. Leatherface is flaying her coworker from the radio station, LG. Here, Stretch represents the power of the gaze as she watches the horror scene; she is very literally a stand-in for the spectator in the movie theater who also peers over bodies to get a peek at some awful and unwatchable image upon the screen. As Leatherface removes LG's skin, and specifically his face, Stretch gags but does not puke, again miming the possible reactions of the horror viewer. Next, she makes a noise that Leatherface hears, attracting his attention. Leatherface has just removed LG's face and he holds it up to the light in triumph before he comes over to investigate the noise.

This moment, I believe, the moment of "face off," represents a paradigmatic, almost generic, moment in horror film — the moment where the inside and outside are revealed at one and the same time and when the permeable membrane between inside and outside becomes a metaphor for the movie screen itself. As LG's face is lit up by the light shining through it, the horror of this vision represents the monstrous instability of surface that defines the relation between representation and reality in the horror genre. The spectator, furthermore, feels fear as an ever receding boundary between fantasy and reality.

In the action that follows the face off, Leatherface actually brings the "mask" of LG over to Stretch and makes her wear it. Ostensibly, he offers her a disguise, a hiding place (a hide), but his gesture is still much more than that; the "facing" of Stretch for Leatherface is a weird courting ritual which he plays upon by next asking her to dance with him while wearing the face. With her new face, Stretch becomes another leatherface and as such she incites anew Leatherface's desire. Also, obviously, in LG's face her gender becomes ambiguous — she is not male here, this is not simply a homoerotic display of desire, rather she becomes literally a "stretch" between genders. LG's face is stretched across her own, her gender is stretched between her mask, her location, her body, and her relation to her monstrous dance partner. Gender, *Chain-*

saw 2 suggests, is skin, leather, face, not body, not internal mechanics, certainly not genitalia. Since Stretch stands in for the spectator, since she has been positioned as the one who watches, the facing scene also puts the horror spectator in the position of seeing through someone else's skin. We literally see through LG (it is his face) but from the position of Stretch. Obviously, this is not simply a case of deciding whether we occupy the male or female gaze; the gaze itself becomes deflected through a series of gender positions, through a cover-up (of Stretch) and an exposure (of LG).

Leatherface, of course, has literally transformed LG into leather which is a different kind of violence, one that uses, rather than simply abuses, the body. Stretch wears LG's face and therefore uses his body parts to create a new space of identity out of violence, a horror identity that will eventually allow her to chain saw the entire Sawyer family. Gender fluctuations in the film are at their most intense at this moment — the mask represents a strange circulation of skin as disguise, as gender, as something that does not fit, as transformative, as metaphor for transformed subject positions from male to female, female to male, victim to murderer.

Quite clearly, what we are watching in this scene are what Jacques-Alain Miller and then Kaja Silverman have called the operations of "suture," or the work involved in cinematic identifications. However, this is suture with a difference because the scene literalizes the operations of suture by emphasizing the transferability of skin and the ways in which identities are sewn into one another. Furthermore, this scene of suture as Gothic horror becomes the narrative itself of a later film, *The Silence of the Lambs*. As we will see in the next chapter, monstrosity and humanity reside at one and the same time in the gendered, raced, and classed skins that monsters and victims take on and off.

In her article on suture, Kaja Silverman summarizes the discussions of suture within Lacanian psychoanalysis and she suggests that the concept of suture has been transferred to cinema studies to ask the following questions: What kind of subjectivities do films produce and presume? "What is the cinematic equivalent for language in the literary text?" "What is cinematic syntax?"[11] The answer, of course, is the cinematic apparatus — interlocking shots, cuts, sweeps, pans, long shots, close-ups, overheads, angled shots — all of which form a language/grammar through which the content of the film is given structure or rendered symbolic. Because she is working within a clearly psychoanalytic frame of reference, Silverman uses "suture" to identify the relationship between lack or loss and subjectivity within the activity of spectatorship. Because there is always something we are denied access to upon the screen, always a perspective that cannot be rendered, a shot that reveals only the limitations of vision, then, she argues, it is lack that structures our relation to cinematic knowledge. Paraphrasing Jean-Pierre Oudart she writes: "A complex signifying chain is introduced in place of the lack which can never be made good, suturing over the wound of castration with narrative. However, it is only by inflicting the wound to begin with that the viewing subject can be made to want the restorative of meaning and narrative" (221). The spectator, in other words, experiences suture first by acknowledging a wound and then by ignoring the wound by allowing the narrative to cover the wound with fiction, a fiction that the spectator must utterly believe in. Once sutured to the cinematic image, the spectator may now endure other camera operations that reveal the incompleteness of vision. Cutting, for example, according to Silverman, reveals "not merely that the camera is incapable of showing us everything at once, but that it does not wish to do so" (222). Cutting obviously both enacts castration and suture at one and the same time.

The ways in which the spectator makes up for lack/castration/not knowing or seeing all, Silverman argues, is to perform all kinds of intellectual, visual, and linguistic acrobatics to make him- or herself feel whole, to cover over lack. Also, the film itself attempts to suture its own gaps and present itself as complete. In classic film the sutures should remain invisible. In horror film, however, we might argue, suture precisely appears as a surface effect and the film constantly attempts to call our attention to cinematic production, its failures and its excesses. Horror film, in other words, is a critical genre and one that exposes the theatricality of identity because it makes specular precisely those images of loss, lack, penetration, violence that other films attempt to cover up. In fact, the excessive specularity of the horror genre challenges the terms and functions of psychoanalytic formulations altogether. Castration, for example, is not the most dreaded event within a horror film; in fact, it is often already a part of the monster's hideous aspect. A monster has repeatedly lost limbs and often he has drawn new strength from such losses. In *A Nightmare on Elm Street,* Freddy Krueger actually slices off one of his own fingers as if to demonstrate his powers of recuperation. In *Chainsaw 2* Chop Top's monstrosity depends upon the visibility of his various castration wounds. For these reasons we have to reread suture as it applies to horror and particularly as it applies to the slasher genre.

Psychoanalytic film criticism, furthermore, seems to stumble over the horror film and possibly over all extreme film genres because its codes of gender and sexuality are too narrow to actually account for what happens in the films themselves. The films, in other words, are more complicated than the theory. In an extended critique of psychoanalytic theories of the gaze, Steven Shaviro gives a convincing account of why it is that "psychoanalysis seem(s) so unsatisfactory today."[12] Shaviro suggests that while "Freud's theories are the very best model we have for the deployment of sexuality under advanced capitalism" (68), at the same time "psychoanalysis is never part of the solution, but always part of the problem. To change the nature of sexual relations in our society it is necessary to *think* them differently" (69). Precisely because horror film is a genre that thinks about sexual relations differently, it has been remarkably resistant to psychoanalytic readings. Shaviro claims that one reason for the inapplicability of psychoanalysis to horror is the humanist thrust of psychoanalysis that implicitly believes that "our desires are primarily ones for possession, plenitude, stability and reassurance" (54). In Gothic horror pleasure often resides in abjection, loss, revulsion, dread, and violence. The abject gaze, the gaze that consumes violence and gore as pleasure, is theoretically inexplicable within psychoanalysis.

It is also worth noting that the monster is not well explained by the language of castration which presumes an economy of lack because very often the monster is the place of excess and fullness. Also, theories of the gaze that reduce spectatorship to the either/or binary of male/female, scopophilic/fetishistic do not respond to the full range of viewing positions available and utilized in the context of the horror film. As we have seen already, the subject position defined by Stretch wearing LG's face and dancing with Leatherface is very difficult to pin down using only psychoanalytic terms; psychoanalytic tools are simply not calibrated finely enough for the intricacies of body horror.

Another example of how suture works (or does not work) in the slasher genre can be found in Michael Powell's classic horror film *Peeping Tom* (1968). In this film a photographer called Mark closes in on women with a camera that has a hidden blade. He then murders the women while filming them, and, to add a final twist, they watch their own death in a mirror placed upon the camera. His object, he says, is to capture precisely the look of horror that the women register when they see themselves being seen and murdered at the same time. Mark works on the side as a soft pornographer; he makes "views" of call girls for other men to look at but he seems to take no pleasure in it. A major theme in this film, and in many of the horror films which followed it, is that violence replaces sexuality as a primary source of pleasure. The pleasure is seeing/violating not seeing/fucking. Very rarely is rape the object. Penetration is associated with weapons not penises — as Clover claims, these weapons are phallic and yet they are *not* penises. In this film the camera is the weapon/penis/masturbatory object, in other films it will be chain saws or blades.

As he is photographing women one day, Mark comes across a model with a harelip and suddenly becomes excited — the gaze in the horror film seems to love and seek out deformity and imperfection. Suddenly, the harelip represents the realm of the pornographic for Mark not only because it is closer to the "real" but also because it is a "mark" of past violation, a place where another weapon has previously penetrated the body and left its scar. Also, we notice that the harelip has been messed with, sutured — it looks like a wound, a place that has been penetrated and bears the scar. In horror film pleasure resides in the visibility of suture, the wound that has been barely covered over because the mark represents the place where the inside threatens to show through. This moment in *Peeping Tom* is kin to the flayed face scene in *Chainsaw 2* and, as we see in the next chapter, it becomes the motivating theme in *The Silence of the Lambs*. There is also a face-ripping scene in *A Nightmare on Elm Street* when the first female victim of Freddy Krueger reaches up to touch the monster and his face comes off in her hand, and another in *Halloween* (1978) when Laurie (Jamie Lee Curtis) pulls the skinlike Halloween mask off of Michael Myers's face. Taking off or stripping in horror usually refers to skin not clothes. The harelip is the mark of disclosure, the potential "opening up" of the body, as Clover has put it. The camera, like the chain saw, wants to see what's underneath and is constantly drawn to the places where the skin appears to give way.

Obviously, the harelip is overdetermined in this scene. The woman's mouth stands in for (in Freudian terms, represents a displacement upwards of) the female genitalia; but the lips are labial and vaginal rather than simply labia and vagina. Similarly, the camera is phallic and penile but it is not a penis. The stakes in this distinction are crucial to an understanding of the horror genre and its symbolic cycles. I have been arguing that skin represents manipulated gender in slasher films and its fragility emblematizes the unstable boundary between representation and reality that horror plays with. Furthermore, the horror film makes visible the marks of suture that classic realism attempts to cover up. This suggests that metaphoricity itself within the horror genre remains intensely problematic. As I suggested earlier in relation to the vampire narrative, the vampire is a figure for both a metaphoricity gone wild (it represents too much) and for the loss of metaphoricity (it represents only itself). How does the slasher film use metaphors?

In slasher horror film, violence is the act performed by men upon female bodies in ways which sometimes make the violence into a metaphor for sexuality but more often the violence represents violence itself and nothing more; mostly, in fact, the chain sawing or the knifing *is* the desired activity. In one genre, rape revenge, as Clover points out, the films seem to "require a real penis and a real orifice" (157). But this does not mean that, while previously sex was metaphorized through violence, now it is *literalized* as sex but rather we must say that the penis and the vagina are stand-ins for the chain saw and skin. This is to reverse the relationship between the vehicle and the tenor—within this system of meaning, chain saw and skin are primary markers of identity and penis and vagina are simply secondary representations. Rape, in other words, is not the sexual enactment of violence; it is still a violence but it is a violence enacted with bodily or fleshly weapons. *Sex is a metaphor for violence* and not the other way round.

Clover does not necessarily agree, she says, rather, that in the realm of rape revenge, "gender is primary and sex is secondary" so that raped bodies are feminine and rapers are masculine and this allows for the fluctuations of male gazes. Clover, of course, has invested in arguing for a gender cross-identification between male viewers and female bodies. This allows her to propose a more complicated version of spectatorship than the ones which assume men watch rapes and then do them. But it also allows her to ignore the empowerment of female viewers and the fear of male viewers. If we argue that sex is a metaphor for violence and not the other way round, then we can deessentialize the relations between men and women and violence and see the possibility of a female violence connected to female visual pleasure and male terror. In other words, while women cannot (easily) obtain penises, they can and do pick up chain saws, knives, guns, and ice picks.

To return, then, to the operation of metaphoricity within the horror film, I am resisting a theory of metaphor that makes violence a thinly veiled metaphor for male-on-female rape and I am suggesting that skin in slasher films represents the blurred boundary between representation and the real. Shots of skin in horror film—the harelip, the cut, the torn or flayed hide—these are metonymy for the uncovering of a psychic wound that *cannot always be sutured.* Classic cinema depends upon perfect suture, horror film depends upon showing what has been sutured. The lack of suture or the exposure of suturing within the horror film creates the need for a very different spectator position and new formulations of the gaze.

Skin, furthermore, covers and uncovers new genders. In the wild conclusion to *Chainsaw 2,* Stretch has cornered Chop Top in a cave where the Sawyer grandmother sits mummified in a rocking chair holding a chain saw. After a final face-off, Stretch saws Chop Top and exits the cave waving the chain saw above her head in triumph. Clover describes Stretch's performance here as a drag performance: "Whatever else it may be, Stretch's waving of the chain saw is a moment of high drag. Its purpose is not to make us forget that she is a girl but to thrust that fact upon us" (59). It is important to Clover that we recognize the girlness of Stretch at the same time as we acknowledge her masculinity because it is the bothness of her body that allows her to stand in for the male viewer: "We are, as an audience, in the end 'masculinized' by and through the very figure by and through whom we were earlier 'feminized.' The same body does for both, and that body is female" (59). Again, I would contend that such a reading leaves intact the presumed male spectator and again avoids the possibility of a more radical and possible queer gaze.

A queer reading of this scene, and of the horror film in general, resists the axes of male and female, feminine and masculine, and it demands that horror be read backwards through the history of horror and forwards through the potential of horror. First, the grandmother in the rocking chair directly quotes the Bates mother in Hitchcock's *Psycho* (1960) where her presence registered her son's psychopathology. She represented his gender trouble as based upon his need to occupy the place of the feminine by erasing women. Here, the grandmother armed with chain saws represents a new form of gender trouble—the potent combination that wins out in this scene is chain saw and breasts. The grandma sits with breasts exposed and chain saws crossed over her bosom. It is from this monstrous maternal figure (mammary dentata) that Stretch takes a chain saw and becomes a conqueror. Stretch, who has threatened all along to just be tits and ass, has now become tits and a chain saw or ass and a chain saw and she drives the blade into Chop Top's stomach, literally chopping his top. The chain saw now stands for the chain of signifiers that has become scrambled in the bellylike pit of the Sawyer mansion. Back above ground the DJ plays the tune and Chop Top must sing along. The grandmother is literally a rocker here, a spectator and a listener to the sounds of violence. The grandma, furthermore, is our stand-in as spectator — we too sit in our chairs, possibly more dead than alive; we will Stretch to the final victory; we watch her chain saw rebel yell.

The scrambling of gender identities and performances that marks the narrative progression in *Chainsaw 2* sounds very similar to the rabid degeneration of categories and activities in another slasher-type film, *Rabid* (1977). In an essay called "The Traffic in Leeches: David Cronenberg's *Rabid* and the Semiotics of Parasitism," Ira Livingston precisely outlines the rabid abject in relation to the circulation of meaning through parasitism. Describing the flows and their directions that map out infection within *Rabid*, Livingston writes:

> The mutant woman who comes to occupy the center of the film figures a dazzling confusion between the sites and functions of production, reproduction, and consumption, succinctly condensed into a prohibited exchange of features (or what I have above called "a crisis in location and direction") between breast, mouth and penis (a list which threatens to be extended indefinitely to include umbilicus, vagina, anus, hand, eye, needle, etc.).[13]

In other words, rabidity, in a horror film about chains of infection, maps out a new narrative form, one characterized not by straightforward progression but by cycles of parasitism and regimes of semiotic chaos. Parasitism, for Livingston, represents the reversal and transversals of flows of bodily fluids, power, capital, skin, desire, disease, bullets, violence. What should be consumed becomes a consumer, what should produce sucks, what should penetrate is swallowed alive. Gothicized bodies, within this system, are those criss-crossed by multidirectional axes of infection and identity. The parasitism that characterizes the rabid, moreover, is already present in many other less obviously Gothic sites, such as the family, the hospital, the media, the mall.

Rabid gender, within Livingston's model, becomes a confusing hybrid of many seemingly incompatible features. If Gothic horror, as I have argued earlier in this study, is produced through generic hybridity or when romance collides with thriller collides with self-referentiality, gender horror is produced when female bodies become rabid (as happens in *Rabid*) and grow penises that they use to penetrate those who would penetrate them or when (stretched) girls pick up chain saws and wave them furiously at Chop Tops and Leatherfaces.

We have seen in several films already how skin mutates. In its various signifying forms, skin is a metaphor in horror for the screen, the place where the inside threatens to become the outside, and finally the place of suture that only barely conceals the mess of identity and subjectivity underneath (harelip and leatherface). In *Rabid* Livingston discusses skin as metaphor and metonymy for cash flows and commodity. The original rabid woman, Rose, becomes rabid after a failed cosmetic surgery that grafts artificial skin onto her body to repair damage done to her in a motorcycle accident. The neutralization of the skin tissue before it is grafted represents the logic of capitalism that transforms everything into capital but that also produces the conditions for vengeance, produces its own grave diggers. This again is precisely "the traffic in leeches" or the logic of parasitism — what you eat will eat you. The ambiguous relationship between consumers and producers in horror film plays itself out specifically in the location of the cinema and through the fears of its audiences. The audience precisely worries that what it consumes will later consume it, what it watches will later manifest as a lurking peeping Tom, and what it watches die will later rise again to stalk.

For Livingston the chaos produced by gender horror in *Rabid* is best summarized in a manic shopping mall sequence where rabid bodies circulate infecting innocent shoppers; here sucking and blowing, shooting and penetrating are all scrambled in the exchange of bullets, lights, looks, and words that culminate in what Livingston calls the death of the author when the mall Santa Claus is sprayed with bullets — the giver gets, the circulation of commodities becomes the circulation of violences that masquerade as sex but only long enough to strike. Livingston says it best: "Something happened. The glimpses of the cross-functional mechanism weave through the film like a needle through fabric. Each time it is the same — but slightly different" (532).

Each time it is the same but slightly different. Stretch waving her chain saw repeats the ending to *Chainsaw* where Leatherface was left frantically waving his chain saw at his escaping female victim. Leatherface is replaced by Stretch, who has been leatherfaced, and Stretch has subtly altered the flow, the direction, and the location of gender markings by her chain sawing. If we return briefly to the concept of bodies that splatter and Judith Butler's notion of the construction of identity "through exclusionary means," we find that the horror film enacts the violence of naming. As usual in Gothic, the chain saw cuts both ways and the splattering of bodies simultaneously pulverizes otherness *and* sutures it to new and increasingly odd subject positions. If identity in Butler's scheme of what bodies matter seems bound by the binary of girls and boys, no such binary operates in Gothic. In Gothic horror identity is always part of a cycle and as one identity, let's say girl/victim, disappears into the void, another, let's say Stretch with chain saw, rises out of the gore prepared to chisel a new body for herself. Stretch's lethal performance of gender with an edge is not high drag but an intense blast of interference that messes up once and for all the generic identity codes that read femininity into tits and ass and masculinity into penises. The chain saw has been sutured and grafted onto the female body rendering it a queer body of violence and power, a monstrous body that has blades, makes noise, and refuses to splatter.

7

Skinflick: Posthuman Gender in Jonathan

Demme's The Silence of the Lambs

Nor let the beetle, nor the death-moth be
Your mournful Psyche . . .
—*John Keats,* ODE ON MELANCHOLY

Skinflick

The monster, as we know it, died in 1963 when Hannah Arendt published her "Report on the Banality of Evil" entitled *Eichmann in Jerusalem.* Adolf Eichmann, as the representative of a system of unspeakable horror, stood trial for "crimes committed against humanity." Arendt refused, in her report, to grant the power of horror to the ordinary looking man who stood trial. While the press commented on the monster who hides behind the banal appearance, Arendt turned the equation around and recognized the banality of a monstrosity that functions as a bureaucracy. She writes:

> [The prosecutor] wanted to try the most abnormal monster the world had ever seen. . . . [The judges] knew, of course, that it would have been very comforting indeed to believe that Eichmann was a monster, even though if he had been Israel's case against him would have collapsed. . . . The trouble with Eichmann was precisely that so many were like him, and that the many were neither perverted nor sadistic, that they were, and still are, terribly and terrifyingly normal.[1]

Arendt's relegation of Eichmann from monster dripping with the blood of a people to the conformist clerk who does his job and does not ask questions suggests that crime and corrupt politics and murder all demand complicit and silent observers. Eichmann's crime was precisely that he was no monster, he was simply "terrifyingly normal."

What exactly is the comfort of making Eichmann or others like him into monsters? Monsters, as I have been arguing throughout this study, confirm that evil resides only in specific bodies and particular psyches. Monstrosity as the bodily manifestation of evil makes evil into a local effect, not generalizable across a society or culture. But modernity has eliminated the comfort of monsters because we have seen, in Nazi Germany and elsewhere, that evil works often as a system, it works through institutions and it works as a *banal* (meaning "common to all") mechanism. In other words, evil stretches across cultural and political productions as complicity and collaboration and it manifests itself as a seamless norm rather than as some monstrous disruption.

The postmodern condition has variously been theorized as "the politics of appropriation" and "the politics of difference"[2]; as a "cultural logic of late capitalism"[3]; as "a patchwork of overlapping alliances."[4] Donna Haraway, in a crucial essay on feminism and postmodernism, uses the cyborg as a symbol for the fragmentations and alliances that make up a postmodern feminist subjectivity. At one point in the essay, she compares her cyborg to Frankenstein's monster: "Unlike Frankenstein's monster, the cyborg does not expect its father to save it through a restoration of the garden, that is through the fabrication of a heterosexual mate, through its completion in a finished whole, a city and a cosmos."[5] She adds later, "single vision produces worse illusions than double vision or many-headed monsters. Cyborg unities are monstrous and illegitimate" (196). Haraway's invocation of the cyborg subject marks the change within postmodernism of the cultural locations of the human and the monstrous. As she points out, while Frankenstein's monster sought admission to the human community, the cyborg monster celebrates itself as peripheral to family and to the human. The postmodern monster is no longer the hideous other storming the gates of the human citadel, he has already disrupted the careful geography of human self and demon other and he makes the peripheral and the marginal part of the center. Monsters within postmodernism are already inside — the house, the body, the head, the skin, the nation — and they work their way out. Accordingly, it is the human, the facade of the normal, that tends to become the place of terror within postmodern Gothic.

Postmodernity makes monstrosity a function of consent and a result of habit. Monsters of the nineteenth century — like Frankenstein, like

Dracula — certainly still scare and chill but they scare us from a distance. We wear modern monsters like skin, they are us, they are on us and in us. Monstrosity no longer coagulates into a specific body, a single face, a unique feature; it is replaced with a banality that fractures resistance because the enemy becomes harder to locate and looks more like the hero. What were monsters are now facets of identity; the sexual other and the racial other can no longer be safely separated from self. But still, we keep our monsters ready.

Postmodern horror lies just beneath the surface, it lurks in dark alleys, it hides behind a rational science, it buries itself in respectable bodies, so the story goes. In one postmodern horror movie, *The Silence of the Lambs* (1991) by Jonathan Demme, fear no longer assumes a depth/surface model; after this movie (but perhaps all along) horror resides at the level of skin itself. Skin is at once the most fragile of boundaries and the most stable of signifiers; it is the site of entry for the vampire, the signifier of race for the nineteenth-century monster. Skin is precisely what does not fit; Frankenstein sutures his monster's ugly flesh together by binding it in a yellow skin, too tight and too thick. When, in the modern horror movie, terror rises to the surface, the surface itself becomes a complex web of pleasure and danger; the surface rises to the surface, the surface becomes Leatherface, becomes Demme's Buffalo Bill, and everything that rises must converge.

Demme's film weaves its horror and its pleasure around the remains of other horror films and literature. It quotes from Alfred Hitchcock's *Psycho,* from Brian De Palma's *Dressed To Kill,* from William Wyler's *The Collector* and it features a reincarnation of Bram Stoker's insane Renfield, the murderous idiot savant of *Dracula.* This film, indeed, has cannibalized its genre, consumed it bones and all and reproduced it in a slick and glossy representation of representations of violence, murder, mutilation, matricide, and the perverse consequences of gender confusion. *The Silence of the Lambs* is precisely never silent; it hums with past voices and with other stories; it holds the murmur of vampires, the outrage of the monster's articulations, the whispers of the beasts who were told but never got to tell. The viewer is now simultaneously installed as a listener, a listener to the narrative of the monster.

But in *The Silence of the Lambs,* the monster is everywhere and everyone and the monster's story is not distinguishable from other textual productions validated within the film. *The Silence of the Lambs* skillfully pits Jodie Foster as FBI agent Clarice Starling against the charismatic

intellect of ex-psychiatrist and serial murderer Dr. Hannibal "the Cannibal" Lecter played by Anthony Hopkins. Starling goes to visit Lecter
in his maximum security cell in order to engage his help in tracking down
a serial killer. The murderer has been nicknamed Buffalo Bill because he
skins his female victims after murdering them. Starling is no match for
Lecter and he manipulates her by insisting upon "quid pro quo," or an
equal exchange of information. In return for information about Buffalo
Bill, Lecter demands that Starling tell him her nightmares, her most
awful memories of childhood, her darkest fears. As she reveals her stories
to Lecter's scrutiny, Starling is forced to relinquish the authority invested
in her position as detective. Suddenly, with only the glass separating the
two, Starling seems no more free than Lecter, both are incarcerated by
knowledge or lack of, by memory, by power structures, by violence, by
the unnameable menace of Lecter the Intellecter.

Dr. Hannibal Lecter is considered an unusual threat to society not
simply because he murders people and consumes them but because as a
psychiatrist he has access to minds. He is someone "you don't want
inside your head," Starling's boss warns her; of course, you don't want
him inside your body either and you certainly don't want to let him put
you inside his! Boundaries between people (detective and criminal, men
and women, murderers and victims) are all mixed up in this film until they disappear altogether, becoming as transparent as the glass that
(barely) divides Lecter and Starling. Lecter illustrates to perfection the
spooky and uncanny effect of confusing boundaries, inside and outside,
consuming and being consumed, watching and being watched. He spe-
cializes in getting under one's skin, into one's thoughts and he makes
little of the classic body/mind split as he eats bodies and sucks minds dry.

The subplot in *The Silence of the Lambs* involves the tracking of
murderer/mutilator Buffalo Bill. Buffalo Bill, we find out, skins his victims because he suffers a kind of gender dysphoria that he thinks can be
solved by covering himself in female skin; in fact, he is making himself a
female bodysuit, or "a woman suit," as Starling puts it, and he murders
simply to gather the necessary fabric. Buffalo Bill, of course, is no Lecter,
no thinker, he is all body, but the wrong body. Lecter points out that
Buffalo Bill hates identity, he is simply at odds with any identity whatsoever; no body, no gender will do and so he has to sit at home with his
skins and fashion a completely new one. What he constructs is a posthuman gender, a gender beyond the body, beyond the human, and a veritable carnage of identity.

As I noted in the last chapter in relation to Judith Butler's concept of "bodies that matter," the human proceeds from and produces proper forms of gender, race, and sexuality. "We see this most clearly," she writes, "in the examples of those abjected beings who do not appear properly gendered; it is their very humanness that comes into question."[6] Furthermore, improper gender often brushes up against unstable sexuality and invokes a homophobic response. In *The Silence of the Lambs,* the tricky constellation of uncertain gender and improper sex creates the "abjected being" of Buffalo Bill. However, as I will argue in what follows, the cause for Buffalo Bill's extreme violence against women lies not in his gender confusion or his sexual orientation but in his humanist presumption that his sex and his gender and his orientation must all match-up to a mythic norm of white heterosexual masculinity. As we saw in *The Texas Chainsaw Massacre 2,* it is possible, especially within the horror genre, to create new genders and to graft them onto old bodies with powerful results. What Buffalo Bill is about, unfortunately, is the crafting of an old gender from new bodies to wear upon his "posthuman" frame.

Buffalo Bill symbolizes the problem of a kind of literal skin dis-ease but all the other characters in the film are similarly, although not necessarily pathologically, discomforted. Skin, in this movie, creeps and crawls, it is the most fragile of covers and also the most sticky. Skin becomes a metaphor for surface, for the external; it is the place of pleasure and the site of pain; it is the thin sheet that masks bloody horror. But skin is also the movie screen, the destination of the gaze, the place that glows in the dark, the violated site of visual pleasure.

In a by now very influential article, Laura Mulvey writes, "sadism demands a story." "Visual Pleasure and Narrative Cinema," of course, attempts to develop a theory of spectatorship that addresses itself to questions of who finds what pleasurable.[7] Such a question becomes all too pertinent when we consider that audiences change through history even as monsters do. Women were once the willing audience of the literature of horror — Gothic, indeed, was written for female consumers — but now women watch horror films with reluctance and with fear, reluctant to engage with their everyday nightmares of rape and violation, fearful that the screen is only a mirror and that the monster may be sitting next to them as they watch. Films that feature sadistic murderers stalking unsuspecting female victims simply confirm a certain justified paranoia which means that women aren't crazy to be paranoid about rape and murder but rather they are crazy not to be.

In "Visual Pleasure and Narrative Cinema," Mulvey argues that

Hollywood cinema has coded erotic pleasures into immutably patriarchal and sexist forms and therefore she calls for a "new language of
desire that would disrupt the pleasure of a male gaze directed at a female
object" (59). There have been many responses to Mulvey's excessively
neat formula for the increasingly messy business of erotic identification,
including Mulvey's own recasting of the terms of her argument.[8] The
most relevant reformulations of spectatorship take note of the multiple
gendered positions afforded by the gaze and provide a more historically
specific analysis of spectatorship. A less psychoanalytically inflected theory of spectatorship is far less sure of the gender of the gaze. Indeed,
recent discussions of gay and lesbian cinema assume that the gaze is
queer or at least multidimensional.[9]

For the female spectator of the horror movie, pleasure has to do, at
least partly, with identification. Do we identify, in other words, with the
detective or the victim, with the murderer persecuted by his gender
markings or with the disembodied intellect of the imprisoned psychiatrist? This film allows us the pleasure of many different identifications
and refuses to reduce female to a mess of mutilated flesh. The woman
detective, or female dick, alters traditional power relations and changes
completely the usual trajectory of the horror narrative. So does Dr. Hannibal Lecter when he refuses to answer Starling's questions until she has
answered his. His story requires her story and hers depends upon his.
Each role in this narrative is now fraught with violence, with criminality,
with textuality; no role is innocent, no mind is pure, no body impenetra-
ble. Each role demands and produces a narrative, more texts about violence and evil and the terrifying realm of "the normal." Like the skin that
Buffalo Bill attempts to suture into identity, stories in *The Silence of the
Lambs* cover the nakedness of fear and fashion it into horror. The camera
glances at mutilation and then frames it within more stories, more sadism, more silence. The silence of the lambs, of course, is no silence at all
but rather a babble of voices fighting to be heard.

I resist here the temptation to submit Demme's film to a straightforward feminist analysis that would identify the danger of showing mass
audiences an aestheticized version of the serial killing of women. I resist
the temptation to brand the film as homophobic because gender confusion becomes the guilty secret of the madman in the basement. I resist,
indeed, the readings that want to puncture the surface and enter the
misogynist and homophobic unconscious of Buffalo Bill, Hannibal the
Cannibal, and Clarice Starling. This film, indeed, demands that we stay

at the surface and look for places where the surface stretches too thin. We cannot look to the ruptures to reveal the truth of pleasure or the pleasure of truth but we can look to the places where skin becomes transparent and see that nothing is hidden. Gender trouble, indeed, is not the movie's secret, it is a confession that both Starling and Buffalo Bill are all too willing to make.

And yet, the gender trouble that Buffalo Bill represents as he prances around in a wig and plays with a poodle called Precious cannot be simply dismissed. It seems to me that *The Silence of the Lambs* emphasizes that we are at a peculiar time in history, a time when it is becoming impossible to tell the difference between prejudice and its representations, between, then, homophobia and representations of homophobia. In the example of *The Silence of the Lambs,* I would agree with Hannibal Lecter's pronouncement that Buffalo Bill is not reducible to "homosexual" or "transsexual." He is indeed a man at odds with gender identity or sexual identity and his self-presentation is a confused mosaic of signifiers. In the basement scene he resembles a heavy-metal rocker as much as a drag queen and that is precisely the point. He is a man imitating gender, exaggerating gender, and finally attempting to shed his gender in favor of a new skin. Buffalo Bill is prey to the most virulent conditioning heterosexist culture has to offer — he believes that anatomy is destiny.

Again, to return to the false opposition between monstrous and normal, it is worth noting that horror film exploits the deviant often to suggest that the maintenance of anything like a norm comes at a price. An entire night world of deviants must be constructed in order to create a world which makes synonyms of normal and law abiding, to prop up these illusions of the just society; horror film consistently parodies such a notion by depicting the world of normal folk as a world filled with zombies. When *The Silence of the Lambs* was released at the end of the Reagan/Bush era, America had seriously reinvested in such equivalencies as family and normal, pervert and criminal, sexual deviance and disease. A horror film like *The Silence of the Lambs* exploits the eschatology of such a universe and depicts the terror of the norm, with a vengeance.

Another Reagan/Bush era film humorously exposes American Gothic as a function of family values. In *Edward Scissorhands* by Tim Burton, monstrosity emerges as a combination of youth, masculinity, and metallica. The monster, in Burton's version, is an unfinished creature who hides out in his inventor's castle until he is disturbed one day by an Avon saleswoman. Edward Scissorhands is an anatomically correct, human-made man except that huge scissors substitute for Edward's hands and the scissors mark both an identity of sorts and an essential difference; Edward's deformity, in other words, cuts both ways. Edward leaves his castle and goes to live with the Avon woman and her family deep in darkest suburbia, scissorhands and all. But despite all attempts to embrace his new community, Edward remains a threat; he is always and forever marked by his metal hands as, literally, armed and dangerous. Edward's disorder is rather similar to Buffalo Bill's — whatever he touches, he tears; his masculinity somehow always presents a threat to young femininity and yet, rather than depicting this harmful masculinity as a by-product of the violence of heterosexual socialization, both *Edward Scissorhands* and *The Silence of the Lambs* seem to make their monsters effeminate.

A film like *The Silence of the Lambs* creates disagreement not just between those who see it as homophobic and those who don't, but between the lesbian and heterosexual feminists who were thrilled to see a woman cast as a tough detective character and the gay men who felt offended by Buffalo Bill. It also divides sentiment along gender lines. I think *The Silence of the Lambs* is a horror film that, for once, is not designed to scare women; it scares men instead with the image of a fragmented and fragile masculinity, a male body disowning the penis.

Buffalo Bill, we may recall, uses female skin to cover his pathological gender dysphoria. He is a seamstress, a collector of textiles and fabrics, and an artist who fashions death into new life and in so doing he divorces sex from murder. This is a new kind of sex killer. Buffalo Bill is not interested in getting in women, he never rapes them, he simply wants to get them out of a skin that he perceives to be the essence of femaleness. Buffalo Bill reads his desire against his body and realizes that he has the wrong body, at least externally. He is a woman trapped in a man's skin but no transsexual. Hannibal's remark to Starling that this man is not a transsexual and not a homosexual suggests that if he were the first, Buffalo Bill would be simply confused about his genitals, if he were the second, he would be confused about an object choice. Neither is the case.

The "case" is precisely the problem and Buffalo Bill's case becomes Starling's as she tracks him to his sewing room. Buffalo Bill thinks he is not in the wrong body but the wrong skin, an incorrect casing. He is not interested in what lies beneath the skin, for skin is gender for the murderer just as skin, or outward appearance, becomes the fetishized signifier of gender for a heterosexist culture. Buffalo Bill's sewing machine treats gender as an outfit made of natural fibers. Skin becomes the material which can be transformed by the right pattern into a seamless suit. But the violent harvest that precedes Buffalo Bill's domestic enterprise suggests that always behind the making of gender is a bloodied female body cut and measured to the right proportions.

And the case is also Hannibal the Cannibal's for he knows Buffalo Bill as a former case history and he knows what he is doing and why. Hannibal was once Buffalo Bill's psychiatrist, Buffalo Bill was once his case. Hannibal, however, created a monster as an inverted model of his own pathology. Inversion in this film depends upon two terms always and neither one can function as a norm. In *The Silence of the Lambs*, inversion reduces norm and pathology, inside and outside to meaningless categories; there is only pathology and varying degrees of it, only an outside in various forms. Buffalo Bill is an inversion of Hannibal the Cannibal and Hannibal inverts his patient's desire because what Hannibal wants to put inside of himself, Buffalo Bill wants to dress in.

Buffalo Bill is Starling's case and when a new body is found in Clay County, West Virginia, Starling's home state, she flies home with her boss to conduct the autopsy. The corpse laid out on the table, of course, is a double for Starling, the image of what she might have become had she not left home, as Lecter points out, and aspired to greater things. This scene, in many ways, represents a premature climax of the horror in the movie. We see laid out for us exactly what it is that Buffalo Bill does to his victims. Prior to the autopsy, the camera has protected the viewer from close-ups of photographs taken of victims' bodies. Similarly, when Starling is being taken to Lecter, she is shown a photographic image of what Lecter did to a nurse — he attempted to bite her face off. But the image of that hideous unmasking is kept hidden from the viewer. In the autopsy scene, the camera reveals all that it had promised to spare us — it lingers on the green and red flesh, the decayed body with two regular diamonds of flesh cut from its back.

The autopsy scene, indeed, resolves the drama of identification for the female spectator who found herself torn between detective and victim. After this scene the gaze is most definitely Starling's. The narrative has seemed to implicate Starling with the victim by identifying the two women in relation to their backgrounds and ages and so there is some tension as Starling enters the morgue to begin the examination of the body. But Starling quickly establishes the difference between herself and the body in the body bag by setting herself up as an authority. She begins her visual analysis of the corpse and at first, as her voice trembles and her hands shake, as her body gives her away, the camera watches her from a position below the corpse — the spectator is positioned with the victim on the table. "What do you see, Starling?" asks Crawford. "She's not local," she replies, "her ears are pierced three times and there's glitter nail polish. Looks like town to me." Unlike Starling, then, the victim is not a hometown girl. The camera moves now to a position above the body and the gaze of the camera abruptly becomes Starling's gaze as we look down upon a mottled arm rotting and covered with dead leaves and other traces of the river she was hauled out of. Starling's examination of the corpse becomes more sure and the tension of identification between detective and victim is relieved for the moment.

Starling, like the viewer, seemed inclined to look away from the corpse, horrified perhaps by the nakedness of violence so plainly detailed before her. But the corpse finally becomes object, thing, posthuman when Starling looks at a photograph of its teeth and sees something in the throat. Before the photograph, her gaze, like our gaze, begins to linger. Turning back to the corpse moments later, Starling surveys the undignified flesh and, speaking into a tape recorder, she begins to piece the body together, rebuild the mutilated body, and learn what the body has to tell.

The camera itself has done a kind of violence to whatever identity remained upon or within the body — this is no longer a body framing an inner life, the body is merely surface, a picture. The camera has framed the victim in much the same way as Buffalo Bill does as he prepares his lambs for the slaughter. Keeping his victim naked in an old well shaft, he addresses her as "it" when he must talk to her. And the camera also enables Starling to turn the corpse into a case, a case that she must solve even as the victim has become a case that Buffalo Bill will wear. This hideous wake, then, foreshadows the scenes in Buffalo Bill's basement gender factory and the autopsy becomes a site of trauma in terms of the film's narrative about gender — the corpse is no woman, it has been degendered, it is postgender, skinned and fleshed, it has been reified, turned at last into a fiction of the body.

We know from what happened to Buffalo Bill that Hannibal's patients go on to lead illustrious careers and so it is an ominous finale in the movie when Starling, Lecter's fledgling patient and the FBI's fledgling agent, steps up to accept her graduation certificate from the FBI; different degree, same profession — crime. As a camera captures her moment of graduation, the flash bulb is reminiscent of that earlier moment, that prior photograph of the victim's teeth in the autopsy lab. As she becomes a "real" agent, Starling is framed as victim, as a lamb in wolf's clothing. As if to capitalize on the decline of Starling's authority, a phone call interrupts her graduation celebration. It is from the now escaped Hannibal, he tells her not to worry, he will not pursue her. The scene shows Hannibal on a Caribbean isle watching his psychiatrist from his prison days. Hannibal tells Starling, "I'm having an old friend for dinner," and he adjusts his clothes elegantly. Hannibal is dressed to kill. Buffalo Bill, of course, kills to dress and only one costume will do.

Hannibal Lecter feeds upon both flesh and fiction. He needs Starling's stories as much as he needs to track down his next victim. "Quid pro quo," he tells Starling; he wants a fair rate of exchange. Hannibal demands that no one be innocent and Starling must have a story to match the story he will sell her. Starling's story is a fiction of her power which is revealed in the process as no power at all but only the difference between two sides of the glass. Hannibal determines the limits of a carceral system. He is not disciplined by his imprisonment nor punished because as long as there are people around him he can cannibalize their stories. The ever hungry mind, Hannibal analyzes people to death. He whispers all night to the man in the cell next to him and by morning, the man, Multiple Migs, has swallowed his own tongue. Hannibal enacts murders through bars and cages, through minds. Prisons come in all shapes and sizes and while Hannibal's is a restricted area equipped with a screen playing a TV evangelist at high volume, Starling is stuck inside her head, her body, and the disturbing memories that Hannibal insists are not buried far beneath the power suit but quite present at the surface, on the top, visible and readable.

Starling's narrative of her childhood flight from her aunt and uncle's house becomes as terrifying as any other aspect of the horror narrative. The pieces of her past cohere slowly as Hannibal extracts each one surgically and then confronts her with it. The secret of her past that threatened all along to be some nasty story of incest or rape is precisely not sexual. Clarice Starling is the girl who wanted to save the lambs from the slaughter, who could only carry one at a time, and who finally could not support the weight. Clarice Starling is the girl who freed the lambs from the pen and then watched in horror as they refused to leave it. Starling saves others in order to save her own skin.

Hannibal stays imprisoned until there is no longer a story to hear. The installments that Starling gave him of her life maintained his interest just as each new killing maintains the FBI's interest in Buffalo Bill. The serial killing, indeed, like the psychoanalytic session, promises interminable chapters, promises to serialize and to keep one waiting for an ever deferred conclusion. Serial murders have something of a literary quality to them—they appear with a predictable (serial) regularity and each new one creates an expectation; they involve a plot, a consummate villain, and an absolutely pure (because randomly picked) victim; they demand explanation; they demand that a pattern be forced onto what appears to be "desperately random" (as Hannibal Lecter tells Starling). "Sadism demands a story," I noted earlier, quoting Mulvey. And the story that sadism demands is the Gothic story embedded in the heart of a consumer culture *and* the realistic story embedded deep within Gothic culture. Lecter's Gothic sadism demands Starling's benign story; and Starling's innocence demands the Gothic tale that she, as much as Lecter, chooses to tell about a series of "desperately random" killings.

Serial killings, like chapters in a periodical, stand in need of interpretation and their interpreters (like the police, the tabloids, the public, the detective, the psychologist, the critic) produce the story that the bodies cannot tell. Starling and the FBI insist that there be a reason, a concrete explanation for the skinning of women, and Lecter complies but only as long as Starling recognizes that she also is complicit in the narrative, she too must tell and be told. Telling does not mean finding a story in the unconscious that fits, it means inventing the unconscious, and inventing the unconscious so that it can lie well enough to keep up with the fiction of everyday life.

Like some monstrous parody of nineteenth-century Gothic, these two characters mimic vampire and Frankenstein's monster. Franco Moretti describes Shelley's monster and Stoker's vampire as "dynamic, *totalizing,* monsters" who "threaten to live forever, and to conquer the world."[10] Buffalo Bill and Hannibal are also totalizing and each consumes other lives in order to prolong his own. Buffalo Bill combines in one both Frankenstein and the monster; he is the scientist, the creator, and he is the body being formed and sculpted, stitched and fitted. Like Frankenstein, Buffalo Bill must search abroad for the body parts he needs and bring them back to the laboratory. The "filthy workshop of creation" is now a basement sweatshop and new material is stored in a well in the form of a woman who Buffalo Bill is starving out of her skin.

Buffalo Bill, however, is pickier than his predecessor — he demands particular human remains, size 14 to be precise, no one-size-fits-all.

"Is he a vampire?" a policeman asks Starling as she is on her way to pay Hannibal a final visit. "There's no word for what he is," she replies. Of course, he is a vampire and a cannibal, a murderer and a psychopath. He is also a psychiatrist who drains minds before he starts on the bodies and perhaps he makes no distinction between the two. Hannibal is, Starling might have answered, a psychoanalyst, a doctor in the most uncanny of sciences. Freud predicted Hannibal when he noted in "The Uncanny," "Indeed, I should not be surprised to hear that psychoanalysis, which is concerned with laying bare these hidden forces, has itself become uncanny to many people."[11] Hannibal and Buffalo Bill play out the doctor/patient dynamic that has precisely become uncanny, homoerotic (heimoerotic), transferential in the most literal way. Buffalo Bill leaves Hannibal his first victim, an ex-lover, in the form of a severed head. Totem or taboo or something more than oedipal/edible. Not exactly father and son, certainly not a professional relationship, the two "monsters" bond in the business of death and divorce death once and for all from sexuality. Murder is no romance in *The Silence of the Lambs,* it is a lesson in home economics — eating and sewing.

Hannibal the Cannibal and Buffalo Bill are Dr. Jekyll and Mr. Hyde as much as they are Dracula and Frankenstein. Jekyll, of course, produces Hyde from within his own psyche and he cannibalizes him when the pressure is on. Hyde is an incredibly close relative to Buffalo Bill — he too is "hide-bound," trapped in his skin, hidden by his hide and hiding from the law.[12] Like Buffalo Bill, Hyde performs his ritualistic crimes for his other half, he murders for Jekyll, he carouses for Jekyll, he indulges perverse desire for Jekyll. The homoerotic dyad bound to one body, hiding one self in the other, allows one self to feed off the other's strengths and weaknesses. No longer homosexuals, they are simply victims of modern science — psychiatry, a mind fuck.

Criticism has psychologized horror, made it a universal sign of humanity or depravity; horror, supposedly, is what we *all* fear in our oedipal unconscious. It is archetypal and yet individual, a condition of language or separation from the mother, a fragmentation or unspeakable desire. Now, in *The Silence of the Lambs,* horror is psychology, a bad therapeutic relationship, a fine romance between the one who knows and the one who eats, the one who eats and the one who grows skins, the one who castrates and the one who enacts a parody of circumcision.

Psychology is no longer an explanation for horror, it generates horror, it founds its most basic fantasies and demands their enactment in the name of transference and truth.

It is no surprise that psychoanalysis and cinema have replaced fiction as the privileged locus of the horror/pleasure thrill. Psychoanalysis, writes Foucault, is "both a theory of the essential relatedness of the law and desire, and a technique for relieving the effects of the taboo where its rigor makes it pathenogenic."[13] Psychoanalysis uncovers and prohibits and in its prohibition lies the seeds of a desire. The moment of uncovering, of course, the moment when the skin is drawn back, the secrets of the flesh exposed, that moment is cinematic in its linking of seeing and knowing, vision and pleasure, power and punishment. The making visible of bodies, sex, power, and desire provokes a new monstrosity and dares the body to continue its striptease down to the bone. Hannibal Lecter elicits Starling's poor little flashbacks only to demonstrate that stripping the mind is no less a violation than stripping the body and that mind and body are no longer split. Starling's memories are peeled back even as Buffalo Bill prepares his next lamb for the slaughter; and the raw nerve of Starling's memory is as exposed as the corpse that she dissected.

As a curious trademark, Buffalo Bill leaves a cocoon of the death head moth in his victims' throats after he has killed them. Starling first finds one of the cocoons during the postmortem when she notices that something is lodged in the corpse's throat. Later, we discover that Buffalo Bill collects butterflies and hatches moth cocoons. While the skull and crossbones markings on the moth are an obvious standard of the horror genre, the cocoon and the moth symbolize Buffalo Bill's particular pathology. Buffalo Bill and his victims are both cocoon and moth, larva and imago. Buffalo Bill is the cocoon holed up in a basement waiting for his skin to grow, for his beautiful metamorphosis to take place, and he is the moth that lives and breeds in cloths. Lecter calls Buffalo Bill's crime "transformation" — he knows that Buffalo Bill is waiting in the dark for his beautiful gender suit to grow.

Buffalo Bill's victims are also cocoon and moth, they must shed their skins and fly on to death. Or they are the moths, the producers of material. By placing the cocoon in his victims' throats, Buffalo Bill marks the difference between moth and larvae, outside and inside as no difference at all. The cocoon is inside the victims and the victims have shed their cocoons; the covering is internal and outside there is nothing but raw flesh. The blocked throat, of course, symbolizes the silence of the lambs to the slaughter. A woman who has been reduced to a size 14 skin has no voice, no noise coming from inside to be heard outside. The voice, "the grain of the voice," is the last signifier of something internal to the body.

But Hannibal, too, attempts a transformation. In order to escape from his prison cell, Hannibal murders two policemen. He cuts the face off one of them and covers himself with it and dresses in his clothes. When help arrives Hannibal is taken out of the facility on a stretcher. By draping the bloody face over his own, Hannibal tears a leaf out of Buffalo Bill's casebook. Identity again proves to be only skin deep and freedom depends upon appropriate dress. But even when he was in the cage, Hannibal was not bound by his chains, indeed he seemed only to be there because he wanted to be, because he wanted to hear the end of Starling's story. Sitting calmly behind the bars, his hands on his knees, his mouth open, the story of Starling's personal horror issuing from his lips, Hannibal resembles a Francis Bacon "Face." His features are blurred, his flesh resembles meat, and his mouth, open to tell, forms the image of a scream that is felt not heard. But another Bacon painting also provides a fitting backdrop to this baconesque film. His "Figure with Meat" blurs human flesh into animal flesh and makes the slaughterhouse a central image of human apocalypse. The abattoir, of course, was at the center of Starling's childhood nightmare and it becomes the setting for Buffalo Bill's sartorial activities. The figure with meat, in this narrative, is Starling but also Lecter and Buffalo Bill. The horrific human figure sits framed by the dripping flesh of what he will eat, a skinned animal with a recyclable hide, a carcass no longer worth saving.

Like the mythical moth that flutters too close to the flame, Buffalo Bill both covets and fears light. He keeps himself entrapped in the darkness and stalks his victims by night using infrared glasses. Like Buffalo Bill, the viewer of *The Silence of the Lambs* can also see in the dark. In the climactic hunting scene towards the end of the film, when Buffalo Bill plays hide-and-seek with Clarice Starling, the spectator watches through Buffalo Bill's eyes. Clarice's clarity deserts her and again, as she was in relation to Hannibal Lecter, Clarice is reduced to a listener. We see Clarice stumbling around through the infrared of Buffalo Bill's bloody vision. But even as we see with Buffalo Bill, it would not be accurate to say we, as spectators, are simply identified with his murderous gaze. We are, in fact, divided between the gaze of the camera that frames its object (here, it is Starling) into still life or thingness and Starling's blindness that manages to direct a gun straight at the camera. Starling has been framed and blinded but blindness (like silence) has a power all its own. To be blind is to avoid being trapped by appearance, it confers the freedom to look back.[14] Her shot in the dark hits Buffalo Bill and blows out a window, letting the light in. Starling has not only returned the gaze, she has destroyed it and remade it.

As a final point of contact with posthuman gender and the cinematic gaze, I want to examine one more manifestation of transformation in the film. Starling traces her clues to the house of the first murder victim and she goes into the victim's bedroom which has been kept exactly as Frederika left it. The camera looks over Starling's shoulder as she picks over the dead woman's belongings — a jewelry box, a romance novel called *Silken Threads,* a diet book. The room is decorated with butterfly wallpaper, a tailor's dummy, and in the closet hangs material with paper diamonds pinned to it, ready to cut out. In Frederika's room Starling finally realizes Buffalo Bill's sartorial pathology. Later, in Buffalo Bill's basement, the camera again lingers upon the signifiers of the crime — textiles, threads, needles, cocoons, a sewing machine, and tailor's dummies. The two rooms are collapsed into one momentarily as the next victim's screams bleed through from the cellar. Buffalo Bill, of course, has become Frederika just as Frederika has become Buffalo Bill — he wears her, she is upon him, he is inside her. Victim and murderer are folded into each other as Starling enters, gun in hands, to attempt to fix boundaries once and for all.

Buffalo Bill's misidentity forces him to assume what we might call a posthuman gender. He divorces once and for all sex and gender or nature and gender and remakes the human condition as a posthuman bodysuit. Buffalo Bill kills for his clothes and emblematizes the ways in which gender is always posthuman, always a sewing job which stitches identity into a body bag. Skin, in this film, is identity itself rather than the surface of an interior identity. Buffalo Bill, in other words, is a limit case for gender, for identity, and for humanness. He does not understand gender as inherent, innate; he reads it only as a surface effect, a representation, an external attribute engineered into identity. Buffalo Bill is at odds with identity because he is willing to kill to get one; he commits violent acts in order to stabilize his condition. While we are repelled by Buffalo Bill for what he does to women, while the female spectator must ultimately look away from his experimentation, nonetheless Buffalo Bill represents a subtle change in the representation of gender. Not simply murderer/

monster, Buffalo Bill challenges the heterosexist and misogynist constructions of the humanness, the naturalness, the interiority of gender
even as he is victimized by them. He rips gender apart and remakes it
as a suit or a costume, recalling Leatherface's human mask in *The Texas
Chainsaw Massacre 2*. Gender identity for Buffalo Bill is not the transcendent signifier of humanity, it is its most efficient technology.

Hannibal Lecter, with his own masks and dissemblings, is the image
of a violence that cannot be kept in a cage; he is not evil incarnate but
a representation of the evil of psychology; his influence works across
discourse, bodies, and minds, across behaviors, actions, and passivities,
across systems, bureaucracies and institutions. Monstrosity in *The Silence
of the Lambs,* in fact, is always an effect of the surface as it ripples across
fields of criminality, surveillance, and discipline. Monstrosity, in this
film, cannot be limited to a body, even a body that kills in order to
clothe itself, or a body that cannibalizes in order to feed. Monstrosity is
now a disembodied and disembodying force reduced to silence and to
blindness.

Horror is the relation between carcass and history, between flesh
and fiction. The destruction of the boundary between inside and outside
that I have traced here marks a historical shift. *The Silence of the Lambs*
equates history with cannibalism, aesthetic production with a sacralized
meal, Gothic horror with the abject form of that cannibalism leaving
the body. *The Silence of the Lambs* has cannibalized nineteenth-century
Gothic, eaten its monsters alive, and thrown them up onto the screen.
The undead, the monsters who threaten to live forever, find eternal life in
the circularity of consumption and production that characterizes Hollywood cinema.

Conclusion: Serial Killing

Those who go beneath the surface do so
at their own peril.
— *Oscar Wilde*, The Picture of Dorian Gray

In order to close up shop on this Gothic skin show of monstrosity and identity, I want to look at a particular rhetorical device employed repeatedly within both nineteenth-century Gothic novels and twentieth-century Gothic cinema — the pun. Puns litter Gothic horror as if to provide some light (very light) relief to the dark dramas of blood and mutilation. *Dracula* is saturated with puns which make it almost impossible to discuss the text without creating one's own play upon words like "stake," "bite," "fangs," etc. In *Dr. Jekyll and Mr. Hyde*, Hyde's hide is precisely the bleak joke upon which the novel's preoccupation with monstrosity turns. In Oscar Wilde's *The Picture of Dorian Gray*, of course, witty repartee often pivots upon the pun. In many splatter films, and particularly in *The Texas Chainsaw Massacre* movies, cannibalism works like a pun upon capitalism. As we saw, in *The Silence of the Lambs* the jokes and puns are everywhere and they are not only self-referential: they tend to refer to the entire Gothic genre.

Punning involves a particular economy of meaning — it makes use of the same word to express many different meanings which then play off, against, and through each other. A pun, according to the Oxford English Dictionary, is "the humorous use of a word to suggest different meanings, or of words of same or similar sound with different meanings." The word "pun" comes from the French seventeenth-century word "pundigron" meaning "a fanciful formation." The pun, then, is the production of difference through playful repetition. To give a preliminary example of punning in *The Silence of the Lambs,* Hannibal Lecter constantly puns "taste" as in connoisseurship with "taste" as in cannibalism—he is an aesthete but also a gourmet and the most "savage" of the film's monsters (in his gorefest in the cage scene, a copy of *Bon Appetit* is subtly placed in his cell). The Gothic economy of the pun works by making one word or one concept—taste—play across a whole register of meanings. The pun demands that the domestic, the Gothic, the sentimental, and the horrific all exist upon the same surface and that they work through and alongside each other.

Gothic, as we saw in the last chapter, is the production of difference through a repetition of sameness. *The Silence of the Lambs,* in fact, is the perfect place to end a summary of representations of Gothic identities within Gothic horror because, as I pointed out in my last chapter, it has literally consumed entire genres of horror films and reproduced them in "serial form." *The Silence of the Lambs* is saturated with puns to the point that one can hardly discuss the film without participating in them.[1] Visual puns in *Silence* include Buffalo Bill's infrared glasses as puns on the spectatorial gaze—he can see in the dark just as the audience can and as Clarice Starling cannot. This pun on the gaze establishes a rather uncomfortable connection between the gaze of the spectator and the gaze of the murderer. Other appearances in the film of cameras and photographs suggest the technology of the gaze; interestingly, cameras and photographs tend to silence rather than render visible the victims. Skin, in the film, obviously puns on the screen and all permeable surfaces.

A theoretical pun in *The Silence of the Lambs* works through the imagery of patterns—Buffalo Bill and his first victim are linked through their use of dress patterns but they are also connected by the patterns on the police maps that attempt to track the killings. These patterns are described as "desperately random" and therefore not random at all but very precise like a pattern for a dress. We notice how one thing slips into its opposite when it becomes too extreme—too random quickly becomes the equivalent of too ordered. This tendency within Gothic of one thing to slip into its opposite (Buffalo Bill trying to slip into a female skin for example, Dracula's aristocratic bearing threatening to slip into a threat of mass culture) makes mincemeat of any notion of binaries. This is one of the reasons that it becomes so difficult to pinpoint the political impetus of any given Gothic text but it also is what produces the multiple web of interpretations that mark Gothic as both highly readable and unreadable. Gothic puns, at any rate, severely scramble categories like taste, romance, domesticity so that they no longer have opposites. Without the familiar binary codes, the codes that a system like psychoanalysis depends upon for example, meaning itself becomes monstrous.

Puns work at the surface. They posit a surface relation but absolutely eschew a depth relation. I propose that a film like *The Silence of the Lambs* demands that we stay at the surface and it constantly warns against digging deep. Lecter, in fact, tells Starling, "Look deep within yourself," which sounds like a moral or humanist imperative to find truth within but turns out to be only directions to a storage company, "Your Self Storage," which is holding Lecter's possessions, his memories, in a kind of garage space. The garage space is difficult for Starling to get into, the door sticks and she has to jack it up and crawl under. Her method of entry suggests that if the space is to be read as a metaphor of the unconscious, the unconscious is no longer a subterranean vault accessed only through precise and specialized methods, rather it is an unseemly cavern that one breaks into. Significantly, Starling finds something other than what she was looking for in the storage space — she expected to find a body but instead finds a head. This discovery creates a *mise en abyme* effect since the literal head is located inside "Your Self," the site of Hannibal Lecter's memories and subconscious life.

Punning creates or enacts a form of cultural remembering. The punning in this film creates a web of intertextual references that eventually provides a film history traced back not through classic cinema but through Gothic horror itself. We can use *The Silence of the Lambs,* for example, to replay each text we have examined in this study. *The Silence of the Lambs* certainly replays the drama of *Frankenstein.* As I noted in "Skinflick," Buffalo Bill is very much a *Frankenstein* figure working away in his basement attempting to create new life. Dr. Frankenstein precisely took skin and organs from corpses in order to create a new being, a monstrous being of his own creation. While Dr. Frankenstein saw his creation as separate from himself, Buffalo Bill actually builds his monster upon the skeleton scaffold of his own body.

Buffalo Bill and Hannibal Lecter precisely resemble Dr. Jekyll and Mr. Hyde or Dorian Gray and his portrait. Obviously, Buffalo Bill *is* Mr. Hyde attempting to become Ms. Hyde; he also peculiarly resembles the paranoid Dr. Schreber with his visions of feminine metamorphosis. Buffalo Bill hides in his basement and has hides in his basement; he recognizes skin as the site of identity and its reconstructions. Buffalo Bill's creation also duplicates the canvas upon which the portrait of Dorian Gray ages, withers, and grows ugly. His skin has become a canvas, his art is now the art of sewing rather than painting but close resemblance is still the desired object.

Like Mr. Hyde, like Dracula, like Dr. Schreber, like the picture of
Dorian Gray, Buffalo Bill requires a humanized double in order to signify as monstrous. In *The Silence of the Lambs* that double appears to be
Hannibal Lecter although his humanity has been compromised by a
kind of civilized taste for murder. A better double for Buffalo Bill actually
is Dr. Chilton, the creepy psychiatrist who actually believes in psychology and surfaces and depths. Lecter represents a new form of monstrosity, a posthuman monstrosity that ceases to be governed by strict moral
codes of good and evil. Dr. Chilton obviously doubles Dr. Jekyll, Dr.
Freud, and Basil Hallward. He is the scientist, the psychoanalyst, and a
kind of flawed aesthete. Here, finally, we see how science and psychoanalysis and art depend upon the production of monsters in order that
they might verify the existence of something like the human. The relation between the dyad monster and human is always vampiric, parasitical
with the one ever buried within the other.

More obviously, *The Silence of the Lambs* obsessively replays other
horror films. Like *Peeping Tom, The Silence of the Lambs* uses horror as a
joke about the pleasure and danger of looking. Mark is, of course, a
seemingly more benign version of Buffalo Bill; he doesn't skin anyone
but he does slash them and silence them (he cuts their throats) and takes
their surface from them by filming them at the moment of death. Mark
makes his victims' surfaces into a film he can screen; Buffalo Bill makes
his victims' surfaces into a skin he can wear. We recall the eerie moment
in *Peeping Tom* when Mark projects a film onto the back of the blind
woman — her body literally becomes his screen and the unseeing female
is a place that simply holds the gaze that he projects. Female paranoia, we
speculated, was the correct response and one that allows for a blind
woman to look back. A similar moment occurs in *The Silence of the Lambs*
when Starling returns the gaze by shooting into the darkness and hitting
both Buffalo Bill and a basement window that lets in the light.

The harelipped woman in *Peeping Tom* resonates with the various
photos in *The Silence of the Lambs* of Buffalo Bill's victims that fascinate
the police. The pictures are of women with pieces of skin removed from
their backs. The camera, in both cases, always wants to see underneath
and this becomes almost a definition of horror cinema — the desire and
the danger of looking underneath the skin. This desire/danger, as we
know, is replayed again and again and reversed in the paradigmatic horror moment where a face is placed upon a face.

The Silence of the Lambs also replays *The Birds* through the dependence in each film upon fear inspired by noise; we are able to relate the clicking of the shutter in the case of female paranoia to the flutter of the birds and the noise of their wings and beaks. In *The Birds* protection from noise becomes all important but silence is not always the comfortable response — it is usually the prelude to an attack. In *The Silence of the Lambs,* noise similarly works to stimulate fear. Lecter listens, for example, as Starling tells; Multiple Miggs listens and then eats his tongue; Starling listens to Buffalo Bill as she wanders around in the dark and while Catherine's screams puncture the walls between them. Starling has to rely on her ability to distinguish the sound of Buffalo Bill from the sounds of his victim. Also moths flutter around in the basement, directly quoting the catastrophic scene in *The Birds* where birds flutter around in the attic as a prelude to the terrifying attack upon Tippi Hedrun. The image of flying things in an enclosed space produces intense claustrophobia in the viewer and reminds us of the captivity of the movie theater.

Obviously, *The Silence of the Lambs* puns *The Texas Chainsaw Massacre* movies in terms of its discourse on skin, cannibalism, class, regionality, seriality. These are closely related films which actively feed off each other once you put them into juxtaposition. Both *The Silence of the Lambs* and *Chainsaw* are concerned with what we might call the "art of death" — recycling in both films transforms bloody murder into art or ornamentation. In *Chainsaw* the Sawyers transformed body parts into household ornaments; this can be compared to Lecter's flaying and displaying of the police officer in *Silence* as a kind of hideous angel of doom.

All of these films, as Clover has discussed, take us to "terrible houses" — in *Chainsaw* the original house of horror is decorated with the trophies of its victims; in *Chainsaw 2* the subterranean hell-hole resembles bowels filled with partially consumed bodies; in *The Silence of the Lambs,* the prison of Lecter, the basement sweatshop of Buffalo Bill are both cell-like places hidden in labyrinthine structures. Lecter's prison is hygienic and orderly, hidden back behind multiple corridors and locked gates; it represents, of course, the mind within a disciplinary regime, assaulted by TV evangelism and deprived of intellectual/artistic stimulation. Lecter, however, is not disciplinable and he consumes everything that comes his way. Buffalo Bill's basement, like the basement in *Chainsaw 2,* reminds one of the lower body. In *Chainsaw 2* the underworld is one big digestive tract that transforms bodies into nourishment. In *The Silence of the Lambs,* the basement is a gender factory where Buffalo Bill transforms bodies into clothing.

Finally, we ended our discussion of *Chainsaw 2* by comparing the systems of signification in this splatter film to the chaotic systems of meaning in David Cronenberg's *Rabid*. The system of signification that literally goes "rabid" in Cronenberg's film is similarly out of control in *The Silence of the Lambs*. In *Rabid* we discussed the multiple exchanges of fluids and the ways in which flows were constantly changing directions (but ultimately tending towards order rather than chaos). Semiotic chaos produces a wild parasitism which makes it difficult to tell who eats whom, whose gaze penetrates whose body, whose body is drained, whose becomes too fluid, whose remains pure, when business eats pleasure or pleasure becomes profit, or when what you eat eats you. This semiotic confusion, or rabidity, is precisely the effect of intensive punning — flows are reversed, meanings run into each other and within the wild economy of horror, excess dominates the form.

At least one reader of serial systems has found the pun to be an inadequate system of tracing connections between various forms of technology. In "Serial Killing (1)" Mark Seitzer examines the modern phenomenon of serial killing by tracing "the forms of repetitive and addictive violence produced, or solicited, by the styles of production and reproduction that make up machine culture."[2] "Serial Killers" makes a compelling case for the connections between addiction, bureaucracy, and repetitive violence in what he is calling the machine culture and he refers, significantly, to the most addictive of Gothic texts, *Dracula,* to argue his case. In relation to *Dracula,* Seitzer looks specifically at Renfield's peculiar addiction to numbers, arithmomania, and he notes:

> By this quantitative accounting of life, what becomes conspicuous are the ways in which numbers, writing, and bodies indicate each other in circular fashion, such that writing and counting, word counts and body counts, figures and masses, mathematical series and serial killing, addictive consumerism and addictive cannibalism are drawn into taut relation — and not least in the body of "The Count" himself (105).

Seitzer cannily links written accounts to bank accounts and finds that the textual and the economic meet in the body of the count, the man who transforms others into his own likeness. But in a note he cautions against making arguments "by way of the analogy or pun" and he argues that such a method "has the effect of invoking without specifying the relays between persons, bodies and forms of technology" (122).

Seitzer, we might note with reference to his comments on "counting" in *Dracula*, has not avoided the pun himself and this is partly because the Gothic text actually demands that one read through the pun.
Seitzer claims that "proceeding by way of analogies immune to differences is troubling not least because it is precisely the violence-inducing
tensions between analogy and cause that traverse these cases of murder
and machine culture" (122). I agree that analogies "immune to difference" might create dangerous likenesses but the alternative to analogical
progression seems to be a kind of deterministic "deep" logic that proceeds through difference (usually sexual difference) and finds grand and
even universal systems of meaning to explain even local phenomena. The
best example of a system based upon such deep logic is, of course, psychoanalysis itself.

Seitzer draws out and sustains a complicated theoretical argument
about technologies of violence that seem to literally swallow up monster
and victim and produce an almost subjectless system of serial killing. At
the center of this system, however, he suggests, we find a barely concealed white bourgeois male anxiety about erasure. The serial murders
respond to and reestablish sexual difference and the difference between
self and other that seemed in doubt. Seitzer posits "an internal connection between what might be called an addiction to self-making or self-
transformation and these maladies of agency and pathologies of will or
motive" (97). Seitzer's essay is an important discussion of the relays
between bureaucracy and machine culture which produce selves and
anxiety about selves side by side.

However, Seitzer's attempt to analyze what we have called the rabidity of meaning in Gothic draws him into a strange argument. In his
reading of *Dracula*, Seitzer examines how the "representation and pro-
cessing of the materials of sexual violence . . . is experienced in machine
culture" (107). He analyzes the way bureaucracy holds the vampire at
bay and he looks closely at what form of erotic violence the vampire
represents. Many readings of vampirism, including the one I advance in
this book, have looked at the way the novel links vampirism and perverse
sexuality or homosexuality. Seitzer grants that homosexual desire has
been identified in the novel as something in need of "correction." But, he
claims, "the real threat here is not a dangerous homosexuality and not an
endangered heterosexuality but the threat of an erotics irreducible to
gendered bodies and gendered persons and without specific relation to
female or male bodies: the panic/thrill of the highly eroticized uncer-

tainty as to the status of identity and sexual identity" (108). What are the stakes (pun intended) of divorcing vampirism from the binary homo-hetero and claiming for the threat of "an erotics irreducible to gendered bodies"? Furthermore, what is "an erotics irreducible to gendered bodies"? Clearly, the real threat in *Dracula is* "a dangerous homosexuality" *and* "an endangered heterosexuality" and, as I have argued, an eroticized ethnicity and class identity. In this paragraph Seitzer opposes the stability of the homo-hetero binary to the "panic/thrill of the highly eroticized uncertainty" and presumes, therefore, that there is an outside to sexual and gender binaries. As I have been arguing throughout *Skin Shows*, Gothic always plays through available categories of identity and transforms the riot of those categories into "real threat," but this is not to say that Gothic accesses some outside to gender, race, sexuality, and class. Uncertainty is always built into binary formulations, usually as part of the debased category; so, for example, homosexuality plays as "eroticized uncertainty" to heterosexuality's stability. Seitzer's argument therefore that the "real threat here is not a dangerous homosexuality and not an endangered heterosexuality" ignores dangerously the realness of gendered and sexualized bodies.

Seitzer goes on in this section to claim that the novel's conclusion (in which the men in the novel are all fathers to the child and the novel is represented as the work of multiple authors) represents an antidote to the "erotics irreducible to human order" in that it is "the *miscegenation* of bodies and machines" (108). The use of the word "miscegenation" here (italicized no less) suggests that the cross fertilization of bodies and machines is way more transgressive than any racial miscegenation might be. As in the balance between homo-hetero binaries and eroticized uncertainty, specific bodies are left out of the formulation. So, if eroticized uncertainty plays against the homo or gender-variant body, so the miscegenation of bodies and machines leaves out the racial body by implying that racial miscegenation is a kind of stabilized threat versus the radical instability of miscegenation between bodies and machines.[3]

Seitzer's tendency to look for a realm of instability beyond categories actually returns him to a world of male monsters and female victims. His Deleuzian model of technoculture can actually restabilize the coordinates of sex and violence in machine culture. A final example of a place in his article where specific bodies are replaced by machine bodies with disastrous effects comes in the section where he moves from a reference to the "wild work" in *Dracula* to "wilding." He writes: "I have in mind here, of course, the recent episode of male anti-female violence that took place in that repository of nature in the heart of the city — Central Park" (110). It is hard to imagine, given the cultural specifics of the Central Park rape, how it can be reduced to an "episode of male anti-female violence" or an event marked by the blurring of nature and city, as opposed to, say, a case of culturally overdetermined black male aggression against white femininity or black urban discontent against white middle-class security. The attempt to find a wide angle in Seitzer's frame of reference forces him to overlook the specific bodies involved in specific acts of violence. African American poet Sapphire complicates the relations between sex, class, race, and gender in her poem about the same incident entitled "Wild Thing." For Sapphire the wilding incident is no simple and contained episode of "male anti-female violence"; she calls upon the voice of the rapist to describe the world he moves in: "My whole world is / black & brown & closed, / till I open it / with a rock / christen it with / blood."[4] A world that is "black & brown & closed" can only be opened with a rock, and this is not to say that, therefore, black-on-white aggression is justifiable but only that the link between blackness and violence in American culture cannot easily be compared to the white bureaucratic violences that Seitzer discusses.

Puns in Gothic horror, I think, actually maintain certain parameters of meaning within a genre that threatens to run wild. If Seitzer's discussion of the "wild work" of Gothic leads him off into a territory beyond the body, puns return us time and time again to specific bodies and to the body as a symbol of the (at least) doubleness of monstrosity. The pun often plays through opposites without necessarily exploding the opposition; rather, the pun multiplies the oppositions and explores the limits of oppositions and finds difference where there seems to be only sameness and sameness within difference.

A recent film about mass murderers or serial killers reveals the danger of losing the playfulness of Gothic and replacing the pun with sincerity. Oliver Stone's *Natural Born Killers* takes an earnest look at violence and plays violence not through the "wild work" of culture but through the naturalness of violence. *Natural Born Killers* pretends to be interested in murder as a part of nature and the mass murderer Mickey Knox at one point opines about the predatory nature of both man and beast. However, at various moments in the narrative, Stone clearly forces linear relations between child abuse and adult violence and incest and murderous impulse. He also heavy-handedly blames television for the production of a generation of serial killers. While one would not want to argue that incest, child abuse, and television had nothing to do with producing violent tendencies, one would also not want to lock up the relationship between these phenomena as cause and effect. Indeed, Stone's film is less linear than he might like if only because the intense visual effects he uses—mostly MTV-influenced techniques like the off-balance camera, pixel vision, or oversaturation of color—actually reproduce the very styles that he suggests cause teen violence.

As is well known by now, Oliver Stone's film originally used a script written by Quentin Tarantino, the master of Gothic comedy. If Tarantino indulges humor to the point of violent farce, Stone avoids it as if he fears undermining the seriousness of his subject. But, as Oscar Wilde warns, "Those who go beneath the surface do so at their own peril." A wild warning indeed and one that Stone and Seitzer would do well to note—beneath the surface lies the humanistic urge to uncover the cause of violence and the way to end it. Violence, like sexuality, too often provokes a moralistic response.

This book, by suggesting the multiple mechanisms within the technology of monsters and by refusing an easy morality of monstrosity versus humanity, begins its own series of interminable productions. Like Frankenstein's "half-finished creature," this monster threatens to never be complete. "So many monsters, so little time" may indeed be an apt epigraph for this entire project. Within this multiplication, I turn to the mathematical progression punned by Mark Seitzer's article—the word "count" appears again and again in the texts I read: accounts, recounts, counter, counterclockwise, Count Dracula even. Renfield's habit of jotting down numbers in a little black book "as though he were focussing some account as the auditors put it" (73) begins to resemble my own methods of accounting. Renfield is busy calculating how much life he has absorbed from the animals he has consumed. Seward, always (like Freud) wondering how much difference there really is between himself and his patient, comments: "How well the man has reasoned; lunatics always do within their scope." Still on the theme of counting, we could point to the Cronenberg horror film *Dead Ringers* in which an artist designs a set of gynecological instruments for Bev, a twin troubled by his double. The instruments are displayed in an art show called "Mathematics in Metal." We might want to add Frankenstein's monster to the exhibit, also Count Dracula and his vampire women, Dr. Jekyll and his hidden Hyde, Dorian Gray and his twin, Leatherface and Chop Top.

Monsters multiply rapidly, just as Dr. Frankenstein feared, but they have always populated cultural and political boundaries despite paranoid attempts to banish them forever. As we have learned from the horror film, monsters may be exiled, beaten, shot, stabbed, obliterated and still they always return; but the returns of monsters are not "like" the return of the repressed: the returns of monsters are always economic. By refusing to make the human into a refuge from monstrosity, this book imagines a posthuman monstrosity that is partial, compromised, messy, and queer.

In *Skin Shows* I have been attempting to show that the violence of representation does not always lie in bloody scenes of carnage or in images of monstrosity. The violence of representation more often works through well-meaning and sincere humanist texts that feel compelled to make the human into some earnest composite of white, bourgeois, Christian heterosexuality. Nowadays, however, the lunatics, as they say, are taking over the asylum. The monsters clearly outnumber the men and posthumanity is upon us.

Notes

1 Parasites and Perverts: An Introduction to Gothic Monstrosity

1 Jean Baudrillard, "The Ecstasy of Communication," in *The Anti-Aesthetic: Essays on Postmodern Culture,* ed. Hal Foster (Port Townsend, Wash.: Bay Press, 1983), 130. Baudrillard writes: "Obscenity begins precisely when there is no more spectacle, no more scene, when all becomes transparence and immediate visibility, when everything is exposed to the harsh and inexorable light of information and communication."

2 Linda Williams, *Hard Core: Power, Pleasure and the "Frenzy of the Visible"* (Berkeley and Los Angeles: University of California Press, 1989).

3 Michel Foucault, *Discipline and Punish: The Birth of the Prison,* trans. Alan Sheridan (New York: Vintage, 1979), 30, 29.

4 See, for example, Edith Birkhead, *The Tale of Terror: A Study of the Gothic Romance* (New York: Russell and Russell, 1963); Montague Summers, *The Gothic Quest: A History of Gothic* (New York: Russell and Russell, 1938); David Punter, *The Literature of Terror: A History of Gothic Fictions from 1765 to the Present Day* (London: Longman, 1980).

5 This term is coined by Marjorie Garber in *Vested Interests: Cross-Dressing and Cultural Anxiety* (New York: Routledge, 1992), 16. In this study of transvestism, Garber suggests that the cross-dresser and the transsexual provoke category crises that are displaced onto the place of gender ambiguity. This argument is useful to the claim that I make that all difference in modernity has been subsumed under the aegis of sexual difference.

6 Most notable, for my purposes, among such studies are Nancy Armstrong's *Desire and Domestic Fiction: A Political History of the Novel* (New York and Oxford: Oxford University Press, 1987) and David A. Miller's *The Novel and the Police* (Berkeley and Los Angeles: University of California Press, 1988).

7 See Michelle A. Masse, *In The Name of Love: Women, Masochism and the Gothic* (Ithaca and London: Cornell University Press, 1992). Masse's study looks at the intersections

of the Gothic novel, masochism, and feminism. Masse writes: "The novels' central concern with masochism does not mean that characters (or women) are masochistic, although many are. Instead, my premise is that what characters in these novels represent, whether through repudiation, doubt, or celebration, is the cultural, psychoanalytic, and fictional expectation that they should be masochistic if they are 'normal' women" (2).

8   See Susan Wolstenholme, *Gothic (Re)Visions: Writing Women as Readers* (Albany, N.Y.: State University of New York Press, 1993). Wolstenholme has a chapter entitled "Exorcising the Mother" and another called "Why Would a Textual Mother Haunt a House Like This?" She writes: "As linguistic structures novels are always inscribed in paternal law; in one sense (a strictly psychoanalytic one), no text can really have a 'mother' because inscription in language implies differentiation from the maternal. But as I have suggested, Gothic-marked narratives always point to the space where the absent mother might be" (151).

Another study of Gothic similarly invests in exclusively familial metaphors for the relations between authors, Gothic novels, and fear or dread. In *Ghosts of the Gothic: Austen, Eliot, & Lawrence* (Princeton, N.J.: Princeton University Press, 1980), Judith Wilt writes: "Dread is the father and mother of the Gothic. Dread begets rage and fright and cruel horror, or awe and worship and shining steadfastness — all of these have human features, but Dread has no face" (5).

9   Ellen Moers, *Literary Women* (London: The Women's Press, 1978).

10 Claire Kahane, "Gothic Mirrors and Feminine Identity," *The Centennial Review* 24 (1980): 43–64.

11 Gilles Deleuze and Félix Guattari, *Anti-Oedipus: Capitalism and Schizophrenia,* trans. Robert Hurley, Mark Seem, and Helen R. Lane, preface by Michel Foucault (Minneapolis: University of Minnesota Press, 1983), 51.

12 Deleuze and Guattari, "The Whole and Its Parts," in *Anti-Oedipus,* 45.

13 Slavoj Žižek, "Grimaces of the Real, or When the Phallus Appears," *October* 58 (fall 1991): 44–68.

14 For more on this see George E. Haggerty, *Gothic Fiction/Gothic Form* (University Park and London: The Pennsylvania State University Press, 1989).

15 Mary Shelley, *Frankenstein or The Modern Prometheus* (1831; reprint, ed. M. K. Joseph, New York and Oxford: Oxford University Press, 1980), 10.

16 See Patrick Bratlinger and Richard Boyle, "The Education of Edward Hyde: Stevenson's 'Gothic Gnome' and the Mass Readership of Late Victorian England," in *100 Years of Dr. Jekyll and Mr. Hyde,* ed. Gordon Hirsch and William Veeder (Chicago: University of Chicago Press, 1988).

17 Max Simon Nordau, *Degeneration* (New York: D. Appleton and Co., 1895).

18 Bram Stoker, "The Censorship of Fiction" *The Nineteenth Century* (September 1908): 481.

19 See the introduction to Oscar Wilde, *The Picture of Dorian Gray* (1891; reprint, ed. and with an introduction by Isobel Murray, Oxford and New York: Oxford University Press, 1981).

20 Eve Kosofsky Sedgwick, *The Coherence of Gothic Conventions* (New York and London: Methuen, 1986), vi.

21 Bram Stoker, *Dracula* (1897; reprint, New York: Bantam, 1981), 18.

22 Robert Louis Stevenson, *The Strange Case of Dr. Jekyll and Mr. Hyde* (1886; reprint, New York: Bantam, 1981), 18.

23 In an article on the influence of Spanish models of nationhood upon English debates of "the Jewish question," Michael Ragussis looks at nineteenth-century novels like *Ivanhoe* and their positioning of questions of nationhood alongside calls for Jewish assimilation: "By depicting the persecution of the Jews at a critical moment in history—the founding of the English nation-state—*Ivanhoe* located 'the Jewish question' at the heart of English national identity" (478). See "The Birth of a Nation in Victorian Culture: The Spanish Inquisition, the Converted Daughter, and the 'Secret Race,'" *Critical Inquiry* 20 (spring 1994): 477–508.

24 See, for example, Henry Arthur Jones, "Middlemen and Parasites," *The New Review* 8 (June 1893): 645–54; and "The Dread of the Jew," *The Spectator* 83 (September 9, 1899): 338–39, where the author discusses references made in popular periodicals of the time to Jews as "a parasitical race with no ideals beyond precious metals." "Parasite" and "degenerate" became coded synonyms for Jews in such literature.

25 See, for example, Richard Marsh, *The Beetle* (1897), in *Victorian Villainies*, ed. Graham Greene and Sir Hugh Greene (New York: Penguin, 1984). For an excellent article on this little-known Gothic text, see Kelly Hurley, " 'The Inner Chambers of All Nameless Sin': *The Beetle*, Gothic Female Sexuality and Oriental Barbarism," in *Virginal Sexuality and Textuality in Victorian Literature*, ed. Lloyd Davis (Albany: State University of New York Press, 1993), 193–213.

26 Benedict Anderson, *Imagined Communities: Reflections on the Origin and Spread of Nationalism* (London and New York: Verso, 1983), 133.

27 Hannah Arendt, *The Origins of Totalitarianism* (New York and London: Harcourt Brace Jovanovich, 1979), 8.

28 For a fascinating and clever account of the production of heterosexuality within capitalism, see Henry Abelove, "Some Speculations on the History of Sexual Intercourse during the Long Eighteenth Century in England," *Genders* 6 (1989): 125–30.

29 Michel Foucault, *The History of Sexuality*, vol. 1, *An Introduction*, trans. Robert Hurley (New York: Vintage, 1980).

30 Julia Kristeva, *Powers of Horror: An Essay on Abjection*, trans. Leon S. Roudiez (New York: Columbia University Press, 1982), 4.

31 Sigmund Freud and Josef Brauer, *Studies on Hysteria* (1893; reprint, trans. and ed. James Strachey, New York: Basic, 1987), 6.

32 See Ann Cvetkovitch, *Mixed Feelings: Feminism, Mass Culture and Victorian Sensationalism* (New Brunswick, N.J.: Rutgers University Press, 1992).

33 As quoted in John McCarty, *Splatter Movies: Breaking the Last Taboo of the Screen* (New York: St. Martin's, 1984), 16.

2 Making Monsters: Mary Shelley's Frankenstein

1 For a thorough discussion of Gothic locations, see Kate Ellis Ferguson, *The Contested Castle: Gothic Novels and the Subversion of Domestic Ideology* (Urbana and Chicago: University of Illinois Press, 1989).

2 Franco Moretti, *Signs Taken for Wonders: Essays in the Sociology of Literary Forms*, trans. Susan Fischer, David Forgacs, and David Miller (London: Verso, 1983), 84.

3   Marie-Helene Huet, *Monstrous Imagination* (Cambridge, Mass. and London: Harvard University Press, 1993), 126. Huet traces a fascinating history of the relationship between monstrous births and monstrous thoughts from Renaissance theories of monstrosity to early-twentieth-century accounts of the golem.

4   Joseph W. Lew, "The Deceptive Other: Mary Shelley's Critique of Orientalism in *Frankenstein*," *Studies in Romanticism* 30, no. 2 (spring 1991): 255–83.

5   For an article which pays particular attention to the discourse of race in *Frankenstein*, see H. L. Malchow, "Frankenstein's Monster and Images of Race," *Past and Present* 139 (May 1993): 90–101.

6   Daniel Cottom, "*Frankenstein* and the Monster of Representation," *Sub-Stance* 28 (1980): 60.

7   Chris Baldick, *In Frankenstein's Shadow: Myth, Monstrosity and Nineteenth-Century Writing* (Oxford and New York: Oxford University Press, 1987), 34.

8   Nancy Armstrong, *Desire and Domestic Fiction: A Political History of the Novel* (New York and Oxford: Oxford University Press, 1987), 204.

9   Eve Kosofsky Sedgwick, *The Coherence of Gothic Conventions* (New York and London: Methuen, 1986), 20.

10 Mary Shelley, *Frankenstein or The Modern Prometheus* (1831; reprint, ed. M. K. Joseph, New York and Oxford: Oxford University Press, 1980), 57. All further references to *Frankenstein* refer to this text.

11 See Sandra Gilbert and Susan Gubar, "Horror's Twin: Mary Shelley's Monstrous Eve," in *The Madwoman in the Attic: The Woman Writer and the Nineteenth-Century Literary Imagination* (New Haven and London: Yale University Press, 1979), 213–47.

12 Michel Foucault, *The History of Sexuality*, vol. 1, *An Introduction*, trans. Robert Hurley (New York: Vintage, 1980), 37.

13 David A. Miller, *The Novel and the Police* (Berkeley and Los Angeles: University of California Press, 1988), x.

14 Anne K. Mellor, *Mary Shelley: Her Life, Her Fiction, Her Monsters* (New York and London: Routledge, 1988), 122.

15 Eve Kosofsky Sedgwick, *Between Men: English Literature and Male Homosocial Desire* (New York: Columbia University Press, 1985), 20.

16 Hannah Arendt, *The Origins of Totalitarianism* (New York and London: Harcourt Brace Jovanovich, 1979), 81.

17 For more on the monstrosity or dirtiness of that which disturbs a pattern, see Mary Douglas, *Purity and Danger: An Analysis of Concepts of Pollution and Taboo* (London: Routledge & Kegan Paul, 1966).

18 This definition of the monster as filthy mass suggests a connection with the Jewish legend of the golem which tells of the construction of a robotlike man of clay by Rabbi Loew. The Rabbi animates the monster by putting a slip of paper with a holy name written upon it into the golem's mouth. When the holy name is removed from his mouth, the golem returns to a mass of clay. Because the creature cannot speak or think he is called "golem" meaning "shapeless mass" and is considered to be soulless. See Gershom Scholem, "The Golem of Prague and the Golem of Rhovet," in *The Messianic Idea in Judaism* (New York: Schocken, 1971), 335–40.

19 Peter Brooks, "Godlike Science / Unhallowed Arts: Language, Nature, and Monstrosity," in *The Endurance of* Frankenstein: *Essays on Mary Shelley's Novel*, ed. George Levine

and U. C. Knoepflmacher (Berkeley and Los Angeles: University of California Press, 1979), 207.

20 Sigmund Freud, "On the Mechanism of Paranoia" (1911); reprinted in *Three Case Histories,* ed. and with an introduction by Philip Rieff (New York: Collier, 1963), 169.

21 Klaus Theweleit, *Male Fantasies,* vol. 1, *Women, Floods, Bodies, History,* trans. Stephen Conway with Erica Carter and Chris Turner (Minneapolis: University of Minnesota Press, 1987), 195.

22 Ellen Moers, *Literary Women* (London: The Women's Press, 1978).

23 Bradford K. Mudge, "The Man With Two Brains: Gothic Novels, Popular Culture, Literary History," *PMLA* 107, no. 1 (January 1992): 96.

24 See Mary K. Patterson Thornburg, *The Monster in the Mirror: Gender and the Sentimental/Gothic Myth in* Frankenstein (Ann Arbor, Mich.: UMI Research Press, 1987). Thornburg sees sentimental and Gothic narratives as two opposing narratives about the stability of family and domesticity. While the sentimental narrative centers upon the family, marriage, and parenthood, the Gothic tale undermines and calls into question all such domestic enterprises. Thornburg calls *Frankenstein* an antisentimental novel.

25 Terry Lovell, *Consuming Fiction* (London: Verso, 1987), 6.

3   Gothic Surface, Gothic Depth: The Subject of Secrecy in Stevenson and Wilde

1 See Patrick Bratlinger and Richard Boyle, "The Education of Edward Hyde: Stevenson's 'Gothic Gnome' and the Mass Readership of Late Victorian England," in *100 Years of Dr. Jekyll and Mr. Hyde,* ed. Gordon Hirsch and William Veeder (Chicago: University of Chicago Press, 1988). Further references appear in the text.

2 Robert Louis Stevenson, *The Strange Case of Dr. Jekyll and Mr. Hyde* (1886; reprint, New York and London: Bantam, 1981), 79. All further references appear in the text.

3 Oscar Wilde, *The Picture of Dorian Gray* (1891; reprint, ed. and with an introduction by Isobel Murray, Oxford and New York: Oxford University Press, 1981), 57. All further references appear in the text.

4 Martin Tropp, *Images of Fear: How Horror Stories Helped Shape Modern Culture (1818–1918)* (Jefferson, N.C.: McFarland and Co., 1990), 110.

5 Rosaline Masson, ed., *I Can Remember Robert Louis Stevenson* (New York: Frederick A. Stokes, 1923), 269.

6 Matthew Arnold, *Culture and Anarchy* (1869; reprint, Cambridge: Cambridge University Press, 1963).

7 See, for example, Edith Birkhead, *The Tale of Terror: A Study of the Gothic Romance* (1921; reprint, New York: Russell and Russell, 1963) or J. M. S. Tompkins, *The Popular Novel in England, 1770–1800* (London, 1932).

8 Terry Lovell comments: "To gain recognition as 'literature' a novel had to make its first appearance in the three-decker library edition." *Consuming Fiction* (London: Verso, 1987), 11.

9 As quoted in Isobel Murray's introduction to *The Picture of Dorian Gray.* One of these reviews was an unsigned piece in the *Daily Chronicle.*

10 *The Selected Letters of Oscar Wilde,* ed. Rupert Hart-Davis (Oxford and New York: Oxford University Press, 1979), 257.

11   Henry James, "Robert Louis Stevenson" (1887), originally published in *The Century Magazine* 35, no. 6 (April 1888); reprinted in *Partial Portraits by Henry James,* with an introduction by Leon Edel (Ann Arbor: University of Michigan Press, 1970), 139.

12   Robert Louis Stevenson, "A Gossip on Romance," *Longman's Magazine* 1, no. 1 (November 1882); reprinted in *Memories and Portraits* (New York: Charles Scribner's Sons, 1910), 229–53.

13   Arthur Symons, "Robert Louis Stevenson" (1894), in *Studies in Prose and Verse* (Dutton, 1904), 77.

14   Richard Dellamora, *Masculine Desire: The Sexual Politics of Victorian Aestheticism* (Chapel Hill and London: University of North Carolina Press, 1990), 198–99.

15   See Ed Cohen, "Writing Gone Wilde: Homoerotic Desire in the Closet of Representation," *PMLA* 102 (October 1987): 801–13; also, Jeff Nunokawa, "Homosexual Desire and the Effacement of the Self in *The Picture of Dorian Gray,*" *American Imago* 19, no. 3 (1992): 311–21.

16   Eve Kosofsky Sedgwick, *Between Men: English Literature and Male Homosocial Desire* (New York: Columbia University Press, 1985), 92.

17   See Rita Felski, "The Counterdiscourse of the Feminine in Three Texts by Wilde, Huysmans, and Sacher-Masoch," *PMLA* 106, no. 5 (October 1991): 1094–105. Felski fully explores the contradictions and complexities of the appropriation of femininity by aesthetes. She challenges the assumption that "this early modernist appropriation of metaphors of femininity was aligned to a feminist project" (1094).

18   Stephen Heath, "Psychopathia Sexualis: Stevenson's *Strange Case*" *Critical Quarterly* 28, nos. 1 and 2: 103–4.

19   Sander L. Gilman, "Sexology, Psychoanalysis, and Degeneration: From a Theory of Race to a Race to Theory," in *Degeneration: The Dark Side of Progress,* ed. J. Edward Chamberlain and Sander L. Gilman (New York: Columbia University Press, 1985), 73.

20   Gordon Hirsch, "*Frankenstein,* Detective Fiction and *Jekyll and Hyde,*" in *100 Years,* ed. Veeder and Hirsch, 241.

21   Michel Foucault, *Discipline and Punish: The Birth of the Prison,* trans. Alan Sheridan (New York: Vintage, 1979).

22   For an excellent study of the construction of normalizing discourses of desire in the French nineteenth-century novel, see Roddy Reid, *Families in Jeopardy* (Palo Alto, Calif.: Stanford University Press, 1994).

23   Hannah Arendt, *The Origins of Totalitarianism* (New York and London: Harcourt Brace Jovanovich, 1979), 173.

24   Virginia Wright Wexman, "Horrors of the Body: Hollywood's Discourse on Beauty and Rouben Mamoulian's *Dr. Jekyll and Mr. Hyde,*" in *100 Years,* ed. Hirsch and Veeder, 288.

25   Count Arthur de Gobineau, *Essai Sur L'Inegalites des Races Humaines* (Paris, 1853).

26   See Leon Poliakov, *The Aryan Myth: A History of Racist and Nationalist Ideas in Europe,* trans. Edmund Howard (New York: Basic, 1971). Poliakov writes of the Aryan-Semite division of the races: "In 1871 Darwin in his *Descent of Man* accepted the classification, though he expressed some doubts about the 'racial unity' of Aryans and Semites" (256).

27   Homi Bhabha, "The Other Question: Difference, Discrimination and the Discourse

of Colonialism," in *Literature, Politics, Theory*, ed. Francis Barker (London and New York: Methuen, 1986), 148.

28   For an excellent essay on precisely the "ways in which the social and the psychic simultaneously refer to one another, and yet are finally not analogous, do not correspond" (60), see Lisa Lowe, "Literary Nomadics in Francophone Allegories of Postcolonialism: Pham Van Ky and Tahar Ben Jelloun," *Yale French Studies* 82 (1993), *Post/Colonial Conditions*, ed. Francoise Lionnet and Ronnie Scharfman: 43–61.

29   Sigmund Freud, "Fetishism" (1927); reprinted in *Sexuality and the Psychology of Love* (New York: Collier, 1963), 215.

30   Donna Haraway, "The Promises of Monsters: A Regenerative Politics for Inappropriate/d Others," in *Cultural Studies*, ed. and with an introduction by Lawrence Grossberg, Cary Nelson, and Paula Treichler (New York and London: Routledge, 1992), 295–337.

4   Technologies of Monstrosity:
Bram Stoker's Dracula

1   Sir Richard Burton, *The Jew, the Gypsy and El Islam*, ed. and with a preface and notes by W. H. Wilkins (London: Hutchinson and Co., 1898). In *The Devil Drives: A Life of Sir Richard Burton* (New York: W. W. Norton and Co., 1967), a generally sympathetic biography of Burton, Fawn Brodie notes that Burton backed up his accusations against the Jewish population of Damascus with no historical evidence whatsoever and he simply "listed a score or so of such murders attributed to Jews from 1010 to 1840" (266)! Burton was unable to find a publisher for his book because the subject matter was considered too inflammatory and libelous. When the book did finally appear (posthumously) in 1898, thanks to the efforts of Burton's biographer and friend W. H. Wilkins, an appendix entitled "Human Sacrifice amongst the Sephardim or Eastern Jews" had been edited out. W. H. Wilkins, in addition to editing Burton's work, was very involved in the debate about Jewish immigration to England in the 1890s. See W. H. Wilkins, "The Immigration of Destitute Foreigners," *National Review* 16 (1890–91): 114–24; "Immigration Troubles of the United States," *Nineteenth Century* 30 (1891): 583–95; "The Italian Aspect," in *The Destitute Alien in Great Britain*, ed. Arnold White (London, 1892): 146–67; *The Alien Invasion* (London, 1892).

2   See Bram Stoker, "The Censorship of Fiction," *The Nineteenth Century* (September 1908). Degenerate writers, he claims, have "in their selfish greed tried to deprave where others had striven to elevate. In the language of the pulpit, they have 'crucified Christ afresh'" (485).

3   AP, "General Mills Puts Bite on Dracula's Neckpiece," *Minneapolis Star and Tribune*, October 17, 1987, sec. B, p. 5. The caption notes that the offensive picture of Dracula on the cereal box came from Bela Lugosi's 1931 portrayal of him in *The House of Dracula*. General Mills responded to the protest by saying that "it had no intention of being antisemitic and would redesign the covers immediately."

4   Michel Foucault, *The History of Sexuality*, vol. 1, *An Introduction*, trans. Robert Hurley (New York: Vintage, 1980), 105–6.

5   See Nancy Armstrong, *Desire and Domestic Fiction: A Political History of the Novel* (New York and Oxford: Oxford University Press, 1987). Armstrong argues convinc-

ingly in this book that "the history of the novel cannot be understood apart from the history of sexuality" (9).

6   In an excellent essay on the way in which "foreignness merges with monstrosity" in *Dracula,* John Allen Stevenson claims that the threat of the vampire is the threat of exogamy, the threat of interracial competition. See "A Vampire in the Mirror: The Sexuality of *Dracula*," *PMLA* 103, no. 2 (March 1988): 139–49.

7   Bram Stoker, *Dracula* (1897; reprint, New York: Bantam, 1981), 235. All further references appear in the text.

8   A wonderfully clever and witty discussion of the technology and modernity of *Dracula* and its participation in the production of mass culture can be found in Jennifer Wicke, "Vampiric Typewriting: *Dracula* and its Media," *ELH* 59 (1992): 469–93. Wicke claims that the vampire Dracula "comprises the techniques of consumption." I am much indebted, as is obvious, to her reading.

9   As quoted in George L. Mosse, *Toward the Final Solution: A History of European Racism* (New York: Howard Fertig, 1978), 156.

10 See Sander L. Gilman, "Sexology, Psychoanalysis, and Degeneration: From a Theory of Race to a Race to Theory," in *Degeneration: The Dark Side of Progress,* ed. J. Edward Chamberlain and Sander L. Gilman (New York: Columbia University Press, 1985). Gilman writes: "Nineteenth century science tried to explain the special quality of the Jew, as perceived by the dominant European society, in terms of a medicalization of the Jew" (87).

11 Cesare Lombroso, introduction to Gina Lombroso Ferrero, *Criminal Man According to the Classifications of Cesare Lombroso* (New York and London: 1911), xv.

12 Foucault, *History of Sexuality,* vol. 1, 118.

13 Michel Foucault, "The Confession of the Flesh," in *Power/Knowledge: Selected Interviews and Other Writings 1972–1977,* ed. Colin Gordon, trans. Colin Gordon, Leo Marshall, John Mepham, and Kate Soper (New York: Pantheon, 1980), 222–24.

14 Sander L. Gilman, *The Jew's Body* (New York and London: Routledge, 1991), 39.

15 In an anti-Semitic tract called *England Under the Jews,* Joseph Banister, a journalist, voiced some of the most paranoid fears directed against an immigrant Jewish population, a population steadily growing in the 1880s and 1890s due to an exodus from Eastern Europe. Banister feared that the Jews would spread "blood and skin diseases" among the general population and he likened them to "rodents, reptiles and insects." Banister, whose book went through several editions, made pointed reference to Jews as parasites, calling them "Yiddish bloodsuckers." Joseph Banister, *England Under the Jews,* 3d ed. (London, 1907), as quoted in Colin Holmes, *Anti-Semitism in British Society, 1876–1939* (New York: Holmes and Meier, 1979).

16 These beliefs are linked to what is commonly known as the blood libel and have a long history in England. See C. Roth, ed., *The Ritual Murder, Libel and the Jew* (London, 1935).

17 See, for example, Henry Arthur Jones, "Middlemen and Parasites," *The New Review* 8 (June 1893): 645–54; and "The Dread of the Jew," *The Spectator* 83 (September 9, 1899): 338–39, where the author discusses contemporary references to Jews as "a parasitical race with no ideals beyond the precious metals."

18 Sander L. Gilman, "The Mad Man as Artist: Medicine, History and Degenerate Art," *Journal of Contemporary History* 20 (1985): 590.

19   Jean-Martin Charcot, *Lecons du Mardi a la Saltpetriere,* 2d ed. (Paris, 1889) as quoted in Jan Goldstein, "The Wandering Jew and the Problem of Psychiatric Anti-Semitism in Fin-de-Siècle France," *Journal of Contemporary History* 20 (1985): 521–52.

20   Goldstein, "Wandering Jew," 543.

21   Sigmund Freud, "The Uncanny" (1919); reprinted in *On Creativity and the Unconscious: Papers on the Psychology of Art, Literature, Love, Religion,* trans. Joan Riviere (New York and London: Harper and Row, 1958), 148.

22   "Homelessness" in relation to the Jews became an issue with particular resonance in England in the 1890s when approximately ten thousand Eastern European Jews fled the Tsar's violence and arrived in England. See Holmes, *Anti-Semitism.*

23   On vampiric sexuality see Carol A. Senf, "*Dracula:* Stoker's Response to the New Woman," *Victorian Studies* 26 (1982); but also Stephanie Demetrakopoulos, "Feminism, Sex Role Exchanges, and Other Subliminal Fantasies in Bram Stoker's *Dracula,*" *Frontiers: A Journal of Women's Studies* 2 (1977); Phyllis Roth, "Suddenly Sexual Women in Bram Stoker's *Dracula,*" *Literature and Psychology* 17 (1977); Judith Wasserman, "Women and Vampires: *Dracula* as a Victorian Novel," *Midwest Quarterly* 18 (1977).

24   Sue-Ellen Case, "Tracking the Vampire," *differences* 3, no. 2 (summer 1991): 9.

25   Christopher Craft, "'Kiss Me With Those Red Lips': Gender and Inversion in Bram Stoker's *Dracula,*" in *Speaking of Gender,* ed. Elaine Showalter (New York: Routledge, 1989).

26   See J. Stevenson, "Vampire in the Mirror."

27   It is worth noting a resemblance between the Bloofer lady and the terms of the blood libel against the Jews.

28   Karl Marx, *Grundrisse: Foundations of the Critique of Political Economy,* trans. Martin Nicolaus (Harmondsworth, 1973), 646.

29   Terry Lovell, *Consuming Fiction* (London: Verso, 1987), 15–16.

30   Franco Moretti, *Signs Taken For Wonders: Essays in the Sociology of Literary Forms,* trans. Susan Fischer, David Forgacs, and David Miller (London: Verso, 1983), 100.

31   The "pound of flesh" scene in *The Merchant of Venice* also connects suggestively with Stoker's *Dracula.* Shylock, after all, is denied his pound of flesh by Portia's stipulation that "in the cutting it, if thou dost shed / One drop of Christian blood, thy lands and goods / Are (by the laws of Venice) confiscate / Unto the state of Venice" (4.1.305–8).

32   In the recent film by Francis Ford Coppola, *Bram Stoker's Dracula,* it must be observed that this Dracula was precisely not Stoker's, not the nineteenth-century vampire, because Coppola turned this equation of humanness and monstrosity around. While I am claiming that Dracula's monstrosity challenges the naturalness of the "human," Coppola tried to illustrate how Dracula's "humanity" (his ability to love and to grieve) always outweighs his monstrous propensities.

5   Reading Counterclockwise: Paranoid Gothic or Gothic Paranoia?

1   Sigmund Freud, "On the Mechanism of Paranoia" (1911); reprinted in *Three Case Histories,* ed. and with an introduction by Philip Rieff (New York: Collier, 1963), 162.

2   Naomi Schor, "Female Paranoia: The Case for Psychoanalytic Feminist Criticism,"
     Yale French Studies 62 (1981): 204. Schor suggests, in this essay, that "female theory is
     clitoral" (212) and the clitoris is "coextensive with the detail."
3   See U. C. Knoepflmacher, "Thoughts on the Aggression of Daughters," in *The En-
     durance of* Frankenstein: *Essays on Mary Shelley's Novel,* ed. George Levine and U. C.
     Knoepflmacher (Berkeley and Los Angeles: University of California Press, 1979), 88–
     119.
4   Sigmund Freud, "Psychoanalytic Notes Upon an Autobiographical Account of a Case
     of Paranoia" (1911); reprinted in Rieff, *Three Case Histories,* 104.
5   Gilles Deleuze and Félix Guattari, *Anti-Oedipus: Capitalism and Schizophrenia,* trans.
     Robert Hurley, Mark Seem, and Helen R. Lane, preface by Michel Foucault (Min-
     neapolis: University of Minnesota Press, 1983), 57.
6   See Saul Friedlander, *Probing the Limits of Representation: Nazism and the Final Solution*
     (Cambridge, Mass.: Harvard University Press, 1992); Richard L. Rubenstein, *Ap-
     proaches to Auschwitz: The Holocaust and Its Legacy* (Atlanta: John Knox, 1987); An-
     nette Insdorf, *Indelible Shadows: Film and the Holocaust* (New York: Vintage, 1983).
     For further discussion on *Schindler's List* see "Spielberg, the Holocaust and Memory:
     Why is *Schindler's List* Different from All the Other Movies? A Debate," *Village Voice,*
     29 March 1994, pp. 24–31.
7   Umberto Eco, *Foucault's Pendulum,* trans. William Weaver (New York: Ballantine,
     1988), 513.
8   Michel Foucault, *Discipline and Punish: The Birth of the Prison,* trans. Alan Sheridan
     (New York: Vintage, 1979), 101.
9   Sigmund Freud, "A Case of Paranoia Running Counter to the Psychoanalytic Theory
     of the Disease" (1915); reprinted in *Sexuality and the Psychology of Love,* ed. Philip Rieff
     (New York: Collier, 1963), 97.
10   Michel Foucault, *The History of Sexuality,* vol. 1, *An Introduction,* trans. Robert Hurley
     (New York: Vintage, 1980) 130.
11   Teresa de Lauretis, "The Violence of Rhetoric," in *Technologies of Gender: Essays on
     Theory, Film and Fiction* (Bloomington: Indiana University Press, 1987), 37.
12   Teresa de Lauretis, *Alice Doesn't: Feminism, Semiotics, Cinema* (Bloomington: Indiana
     University Press, 1984), 141.
13   Kaja Silverman, *The Acoustic Mirror: The Female Voice in Psychoanalysis and Cinema*
     (Bloomington: Indiana University Press, 1988), 16.
14   Laura Mulvey, "Visual Pleasure and Narrative Cinema," in *Feminism and Film Theory,*
     ed. Constance Penley (New York: Routledge, 1988), 57–68.
15   Linda Williams, "When the Woman Looks," in *Re-Visions: Essays in Feminist Film
     Criticism,* ed. Linda Williams, Mary Ann Doane, and Patricia Mellencamp (Frederick,
     Md.: University Publications of America and the American Film Institute, 1986), 87–
     88.
16   Carol Clover, *Men, Women and Chain Saws: Gender in the Modern Horror Film*
     (Princeton, N.J.: Princeton University Press, 1992), 222, 211–12.
17   Raymond Bellour, "Les Oiseaux: analyse d'une sequence," *Cahiers du Cinema* 219
     (1969).
18   Jacqueline Rose, "Paranoia and the Film System," in *Feminism and Film Theory,* ed.
     Jacqueline Rose (New York: Routledge, 1988), 141.

19   Susan Lurie, "The Construction of the 'Castrated Woman' in Psychoanalysis and
      Cinema," *Discourse* 4 (winter 1981–82): 53.
20   Bellour, "Les Oiseaux," 21.

6   Bodies That Splatter: Queers and Chain Saws

1   John McCarty, *Splatter Movies: Breaking the Last Taboo of the Screen* (New York: St.
      Martin's, 1984), 1.
2   Carol Clover, *Men, Women and Chain Saws: Gender in the Modern Horror Film*
      (Princeton, N.J.: Princeton University Press, 1992), 53.
3   Judith Butler, *Bodies That Matter: On the Discursive Limits of "Sex"* (New York and
      London: Routledge, 1993), 8.
4   Linda Williams, "When the Woman Looks," in *Re-Visions: Essays in Feminist Film
      Criticism*, ed. Linda Williams, Mary Ann Doane, and Patricia Mellencamp (Frederick,
      Md.: University Publications of America, 1984), 88.
5   For an excellent anthology about the sex debates and pornography, see Lynn Segal
      and Mary McIntosh, eds., *Sex Exposed: Sexuality and the Pornography Debate* (New
      Brunswick, N.J.: Rutgers University Press, 1993).
6   Robin Wood, "An Introduction to the American Horror Film," in *Movies and Methods*,
      vol. 2, ed. Bill Nichols (Los Angeles and Berkeley: University of California Press,
      1985), 214.
7   Christopher Sharrett, "The Idea of Apocalypse in *The Texas Chainsaw Massacre*," in
      Planks of Reason: Essays on the Horror Film, ed. Barry Keith Grant (Metuchen, N.J. and
      London: The Scarecrow Press, 1984), 256.
8   See Ellen Farley and William K. Knoedelseder Jr., "The Real Texas Chainsaw Mas-
      sacre," in *The Los Angeles Times*, September 5, 1982, calendar sec., 2–7. This article
      examines the history of the film in terms of the attempts to raise money to make it and
      then the scandal that followed its release when the distributors, Bryanston, somehow
      disappeared with the vast profits. Like some legal case in Charles Dickens's Chancery
      (*Bleak House*), numerous suits have since been filed by the makers of *The Texas
      Chainsaw Massacre* attempting to recoup the sizable returns from this ever popular
      cult classic.
9   John McCarty, "Acting in Splatter: The Making of *The Texas Chainsaw Massacre*," in
      Splatter Movies, 95. The interview is with actor Ed Neal.
10   For articles on *The Texas Chainsaw Massacre 2*, see Walter Goodman, "The Screen:
      'Chainsaw 2,' A Sequel," *The New York Times*, August 23, 1986, 9; L. M. Kit Carson,
      "'Saw' Thru," *Film Comment*, August 1986, 9–17; Joe Bob Briggs, "Working on the
      Chain Gang," *Rolling Stone* 482 (September 11, 1986): 35–36.
11   Kaja Silverman, "Suture," in *Narrative, Apparatus, Ideology: A Film Theory Reader*,
      ed. Philip Rosen (New York: Columbia University Press, 1986), 219–35. For other
      articles on suture see Jacques-Alain Miller, "Suture (elements of the logic of the
      signifier)," *Screen* 18, no. 4 (1977–78); Jean-Pierre Oudart, "Cinema and Suture,"
      Screen 18, no. 4 (1977–78); Stephen Heath, "Notes on Suture," *Screen* 18, no. 4
      (1977–78).
12   Steven Shaviro, *The Cinematic Body* (Minneapolis and London: University of Min-
      nesota Press, 1993), 68.

13 Ira Livingston, "The Traffic in Leeches: David Cronenberg's *Rabid* and the Semiotics of Parasitism," *American Imago* 50, no. 4 (winter 1993): 523.

7 *Skinflick: Posthuman Gender in Jonathan Demme's* The Silence of the Lambs

1 Hannah Arendt, *Eichmann in Jerusalem: A Report on the Banality of Evil* (New York: Penguin, 1963), 276.
2 Andrew Ross, introduction to *Universal Abandon: The Politics of Postmodernism* (Minneapolis: University of Minnesota Press), ix, xvi.
3 Fredric Jameson, "Postmodernism, or the Cultural Logic of Late Capitalism," *New Left Review*, no. 146 (July-August 1984): 53–92.
4 Nancy Fraser and Linda J. Nicholson, "Social Criticism Without Philosophy: An Encounter Between Feminism and Postmodernism," in *Feminism/Postmodernism*, ed. Linda J. Nicholson (New York and London: Routledge, 1990), 35.
5 Donna Haraway, "A Manifesto For Cyborgs: Science, Technology and Socialist Feminism in the 1980's," in Nicholson, *Feminism/Postmodernism*, 192.
6 Judith Butler, introduction to *Bodies That Matter: On the Discursive Limits of "Sex"* (New York and London: Routledge, 1993), 8.
7 See Laura Mulvey, "Visual Pleasure and Narrative Cinema," in *Feminism and Film Theory*, ed. Constance Penley (New York: Routledge, 1988), 64.
8 Some of the most interesting rewritings of Mulvey include: Teresa de Lauretis, *Alice Doesn't: Feminism, Semiotics, Cinema* (Bloomington: Indiana University Press, 1984); Mary Ann Doane, "Film and the Masquerade: Theorizing the Female Spectator," *Screen* 23, no. 3/4 (September/October 1982): 74–88; see also Laura Mulvey, "Afterthoughts on 'Visual Pleasure and Narrative Cinema' Inspired by *Duel in the Sun*," in *Feminism and Film Theory*.
9 Valerie Traub creates a queer gaze by suggesting that the male gaze is easily appropriated by a lesbian gaze. See Valerie Traub, "The Ambiguities of 'Lesbian' Viewing Pleasure: The (Dis)Articulations of *Black Widow*," in *Body Guards: The Cultural Politics of Gender Ambiguity*, ed. Julia Epstein and Kristina Straub (New York: Routledge, 1991), 305–28. Judith Mayne conceptualizes the female gaze in terms of "a woman at the keyhole" where "the keyhole represents something of both the vision of the camera and the vision onto the screen." See Judith Mayne, "The Woman at the Keyhole: Women's Cinema and Feminist Criticism," in *Re-Visions: Essays in Feminist Film Criticism*, ed. Linda Williams, Mary Ann Doane, and Patricia Mellencamp (Frederick, Md.: University Publications of America, 1984), 62. See also Teresa de Lauretis, "Sexual Indifference and Lesbian Representation," *Theatre Journal* 40, no. 2 (May 1988): 155–77.
10 Franco Moretti, *Signs Taken For Wonders: Essays in the Sociology of Literary Forms*, trans. Susan Fischer, David Forgacs, and David Miller (London: Verso, 1983), 84–85.
11 Sigmund Freud, "The Uncanny" (1919); reprinted in *On Creativity and the Unconscious: Papers on the Psychology of Art, Literature, Love, Religion*, trans. Joan Riviere (New York and London: Harper and Row, 1958), 151.
12 In the novel *The Silence of the Lambs* by Thomas Harris (New York: St. Martin's, 1988), Buffalo Bill works for a leather company called Mr. Hide.

13 Michel Foucault, *The History of Sexuality*, vol. 1, *An Introduction*, trans. Robert Hurley (New York: Vintage, 1980), 129.

14 As an interesting note on the theme of blindness as a fear blocker, in another film made from a Thomas Harris novel, *Manhunter* (1988), the female would-be victim is also blind and her blindness also aids her in her escape from a murderer. In this film the murderer's predilection is to take posed photographs of his victims after he has killed them. He works in a dark room developing film, furthermore, and this is where he meets the blind woman. Obviously, Harris is making connections between vision and the production of horror — what you cannot see will not hurt you, seems to be the message and the dark is always to the woman's advantage. This may be read as a kind of postmodern rewriting of the feminist slogan "take back the night."

8 Conclusion: Serial Killing

1 See Elizabeth Young, *"The Silence of the Lambs* and the Flaying of Feminist Theory," *Camera Obscura* 27 (September 1991): 4–35. Young puns "flaying" as "somewhere in between fleeing and slaying" (7); later she talks about Lecter's "edible complex" and Starling's status as "agent" — both FBI agent and agent as in active subject. In an article on serial killing, Diana Fuss puns Buffalo Bill's character name, Jamie Gumb, as Jamie Gum. Diana Fuss, "Monsters of Perversion: Jeffrey Dahmer and *The Silence of the Lambs,*" in *Media Spectacles,* ed. by Marjorie Garber, Jann Matlock, and Rebecca L. Walkowitz (New York and London: Routledge, 1993), 195. And of course, in my last chapter I punned Lecter and Intellecter, cases and casings, etc.

2 Mark Seltzer, "Serial Killing (1)," *differences: A Journal of Feminist Cultural Studies* 5, no. 1 (1993): 92.

3 I am indebted to Ira Livingston for his reading of Seltzer's article.

4 Sapphire, "Wild Thing," in *American Dreams* (New York and London: High Risk, 1994), 139–49.

Bibliography

Primary Sources

Beckford, William. *Vathek.* 1786. Reprinted in *Three Gothic Novels,* edited by E. F. Bleiler, 109–253. New York: Dover, 1966.

Bleiler, E. F., ed. *Three Gothic Novels.* New York: Dover, 1966.

Burroughs, William S. *Naked Lunch.* New York: Grove, 1959.

Butler, Samuel. *Erewhon.* 1872. Reprint, London: Penguin, 1983.

Collins, William Wilkie. *The Moonstone.* 1868. Reprint, London: Penguin, 1981.

———. *The Woman in White.* 1860. Reprint, Oxford: Oxford University Press, 1987.

Dickens, Charles. *Oliver Twist.* 1837. Reprint, London: Penguin, 1985.

Godwin, William. *St. Leon.* London: 1850.

Harris, Thomas. *The Silence of the Lambs.* New York: St. Martin's, 1988.

Hoffmann, E. T. A. *The Tales of Hoffmann.* Translated by R. J. Hollingdale. London: Penguin, 1982.

Lewis, Matthew G. *The Monk.* 1796. Reprint, New York: Grove, 1952.

Machen, Arthur. *The Three Imposters.* New York: Knopf, 1923.

Marsh, Richard. *The Beetle.* London: 1897.

Maturin, Charles. *Melmoth the Wanderer.* 1820. Reprint, London: Penguin, 1984.

Meyrink, Gustav. *The Golem.* 1915. Reprint, translated by M. Pemberton with an introduction by Robert Irwin, London: Dedalus, 1985.

Poe, Edgar Allan. *Selected Prose, Poetry and Eureka.* Introduction by W. H. Auden. New York: Holt, Rinehart and Winston, 1950.

Schreber, Daniel Paul. *Memoirs of My Nervous Illness.* Translated, edited, and with an introduction, notes, and discussion by Ida Macalpine and Richard A. Hunter. London: Wm. Dawson & Sons, 1955.

Shakespeare, William. *The Merchant of Venice.* 1597. Reprint, edited by John Russell Brown. The Arden Shakespeare Series. London: Methuen, 1984.

Shelley, Mary. *Frankenstein or The Modern Prometheus.* 1831. Reprint, Oxford: Oxford University Press, 1980.

——. *The Journals of Mary Shelley, 1814–1844.* 2 vols. Paula R. Feldman and Diana Scott-Kilvert, eds. Oxford: Oxford University Press, 1987.

Stevenson, Robert Louis, *The Strange Case of Dr. Jekyll and Mr. Hyde.* 1886. Reprint, New York: Bantam, 1981.

Stoker, Bram. "The Censorship of Fiction." *The Nineteenth Century.* September 1908: 479–87.

——. *Dracula.* 1897. Reprint, New York: Bantam, 1981.

——. *Dracula's Guest.* 1914. Reprint, London: Arrow, 1975.

——. *A Glimpse of America: A Lecture Given at the London Institute, 28th December 1885.* London: Sampson Low, Marston and Co., 1886.

——. *Personal Reminiscences of Henry Irving.* 2 vols. New York: Macmillan and Co., 1906.

Walpole, Horace. *The Castle of Otranto.* 1764. Reprinted in *Three Gothic Novels,* edited by E. F. Bleiler, 1–107. New York: Dover, 1966.

Wilde, Oscar. *The Picture of Dorian Gray.* 1891. Reprint, Oxford: Oxford University Press, 1981.

Films

The Birds. 1963. Directed by Alfred Hitchcock.

Candyman. 1992. Directed by Bernard Rose.

Dressed to Kill. 1980. Directed by Brian De Palma.

Halloween. 1978. Directed by John Carpenter.

Natural Born Killers. 1994. Directed by Oliver Stone.

A Nightmare on Elm Street. 1984. Directed by Wes Craven.

Peeping Tom. 1960. Directed by Michael Powell.

Psycho. 1960. Directed by Alfred Hitchcock.

Rabid. 1977. Directed by David Cronenberg.

The Silence of the Lambs. 1991. Directed by Jonathan Demme.

The Texas Chainsaw Massacre. 1974. Directed by Tobe Hooper.

The Texas Chainsaw Massacre 2. 1986. Directed by Tobe Hooper.

Secondary Sources

Abelove, Henry. "Some Speculations on the History of Sexual Intercourse during the Long Eighteenth Century in England." *Genders* 6 (1989): 125–30.

Adorno, T. W., ed. *The Authoritarian Personality.* New York: Harper and Brothers, 1950.

Alderman, Geoffrey. *London Jewry and London Politics 1889–1986.* London and New York: Routledge, 1989.

Anderson, Benedict. *Imagined Communities: Reflections on the Origin and Spread of Nationalism.* London: Verso, 1983.

Anderson, George K. *The Legend of the Wandering Jew.* Providence, R.I.: Brown University Press, 1965.

Anderson, Stuart. *Race and Rapprochment: Anglo-Saxonism and Anglo-American Relations, 1895–1904.* London and Toronto: Associated University Presses, 1981.

Arendt, Hannah. *Eichmann in Jerusalem: A Report on the Banality of Evil.* New York: Penguin, 1963.

———. *The Origins of Totalitarianism*. New York and London: Harcourt Brace Jovanovich, 1979.

Armstrong, Nancy. *Desire and Domestic Fiction: A Political History of the Novel*. Oxford: Oxford University Press, 1987.

Auerbach, Nina. *Woman and the Demon*. Cambridge, Mass.: Harvard University Press, 1982.

Baldick, Chris. *In Frankenstein's Shadow: Myth, Monstrosity and Nineteenth-Century Writing*. Oxford and New York: Oxford University Press, 1987.

Bentley, C. F. "The Monster in the Bedroom: Sexual Symbolism in Bram Stoker's *Dracula*." *Literature and Psychology* 22, no. 1 (1972).

Birkhead, Edith. *The Tale of Terror: A Study of the Gothic Romance*. 1921. Reprint, New York: Russell and Russell, 1963.

Bloom, Harold, ed. Frankenstein: *Selected Criticism*. New York: Chelsea House, 1987.

Burton, Sir Richard. *The Jew, Gypsy and El Islam*. Edited and with a preface and notes by W. H. Wilkins. London: Hutchinson and Co., 1898.

Butler, Judith. *Bodies That Matter: On the Discursive Limits of "Sex"*. New York and London: Routledge, 1993.

Carter, Margaret, ed. *Dracula: The Vampire and the Critics*. Ann Arbor and London: U.M.I Research Press, 1988.

Chamberlain, J. Edward and Sander L. Gilman. *Degeneration: The Dark Side of Progress*. New York: Columbia University Press, 1985.

Clover, Carol. *Men, Women and Chain Saws: Gender in the Modern Horror Film*. Princeton, N.J.: Princeton University Press, 1992.

Colls, Robert and Philip Dodd, eds. *Englishness: Politics and Culture 1880–1920*. London and Sydney: Croom Helm, 1986.

Craft, Christopher. " 'Kiss Me With Those Red Lips': Gender and Inversion in Bram Stoker's *Dracula*." In *Speaking of Gender*, edited by Elaine Showalter, 216–42. New York and London: Routledge, 1989.

Creed, Barbara. "Horror and the Monstrous-Feminine: An Imaginary Abjection." *Screen* 27, no. 1 (1986).

Cullen, Tom. *The Crimes and Times of Jack the Ripper*. London: Bodley Head, 1965.

Cvetkovich, Ann. *Mixed Feelings: Feminism, Mass Culture and Victorian Sensationalism*. New Brunswick, N.J.: Rutgers University Press, 1992.

DeLamotte, Eugenia C. *Perils of the Night: A Feminist Study of Nineteenth-Century Gothic*. New York and Oxford: Oxford University Press, 1990.

Deleuze, Gilles and Félix Guattari. *Anti-Oedipus: Capitalism and Schizophrenia*. Translated by Robert Hurley, Mark Seem, and Helen R. Lane, with a preface by Michel Foucault. Minneapolis: University of Minnesota Press, 1983.

Dijkstra, Bram. *Idols of Perversity: Fantasies of Feminine Evil in Fin-De-Siècle Culture*. New York and Oxford: Oxford University Press, 1986.

Douglas, Mary. *Purity and Danger: An Analysis of Concepts of Pollution and Taboo*. London: Routledge & Kegan Paul, 1966.

Ellis, Kate Ferguson. *The Contested Castle: Gothic Novels and the Subversion of Domestic Ideology*. Urbana and Chicago: University of Illinois Press, 1989.

Erens, Patricia, ed. *Issues in Feminist Film Criticism*. Bloomington: Indiana University Press, 1990.

Foucault, Michel. *Discipline and Punish: The Birth of the Prison*. Translated by Alan Sheridan. New York: Vintage, 1979.

——. *The History of Sexuality,* Vol. 1, *An Introduction*. Translated by Robert Hurley. New York: Vintage, 1980.

Freud, Sigmund. *Character and Culture*. Edited by Philip Rieff. New York: Macmillan, 1963.

——. "The Uncanny." 1919. Reprinted in *On Creativity and the Unconscious: Papers on the Psychology of Art, Literature, Love, Religion*. Translated by Joan Riviere, 122–61. New York and London: Harper and Row, 1958.

Garber, Marjorie. *Vested Interests: Cross-Dressing and Cultural Anxiety*. New York: Routledge, 1992.

Gilbert, Sandra and Susan Gubar. *The Madwoman in the Attic: The Woman Writer and the Nineteenth-Century Literary Imagination*. New Haven and London: Yale University Press, 1979.

Gilman, Sander L. *Jewish Self-Hatred: Anti-Semitism and the Hidden Language of the Jews*. Baltimore and London: Johns Hopkins University Press, 1986.

——. "The Mad Man as Artist: Medicine, History and Degenerate Art." *Journal of Contemporary History* 20 (1985): 575–97.

Glut, Donald. *The Dracula Book*. Metuchen, N.J.: The Scarecrow Press, 1975.

——. *The Frankenstein Catalog*. Jefferson, N.C. and London: McFarland & Company, 1984.

Goldberg, David Theo, ed. *Anatomy of Racism*. Minneapolis: University of Minnesota Press, 1990.

Goldstein, Jan. "The Wandering Jew and the Problem of Psychiatric Anti-Semitism in Fin-de-Siècle France." *Journal of Contemporary History* 20 (1985): 521–52.

Grant, Barry Keith, ed. *Planks of Reason: Essays on the Horror Film*. Metuchen, N.J. and London: The Scarecrow Press, 1984.

Haggerty, George E. *Gothic Fiction/Gothic Form*. University Park and London: The Pennsylvania State University Press, 1989.

Hatlen, Burton. "The Return of the Repressed/Oppressed in Bram Stoker's *Dracula*." In *Dracula: The Vampire and the Critics*. Edited by Margaret Carter. Ann Arbor and London: U.M.I. Research Press, 1988.

Heller, Terry. *The Delights of Terror: An Aesthetics of the Tale of Terror*. Urbana and Chicago: University of Illinois Press, 1987.

Hirsch, Gordon and William Veeder, eds. *100 Years of Dr. Jeykll and Mr. Hyde* (Chicago: University of Chicago Press, 1988).

Holmes, Colin. *Anti-Semitism in British Society, 1876–1939*. New York: Holmes and Meier, 1979.

Huet, Marie-Helene. *Monstrous Imagination*. Cambridge, Mass. and London: Harvard University Press, 1993.

Hurley, Kelly. " 'The Inner Chambers of All Nameless Sin': *The Beetle,* Gothic Female Sexuality and Oriental Barbarism." In *Virginal Sexuality and Textuality in Victorian Literature,* edited by Lloyd Davis. Albany: State University of New York Press, 1993.

Huyssen, Andreas. *After the Great Divide: Modernism, Mass Culture, Postmodernism*. Bloomington: Indiana University Press, 1986.

Johnson, George. *Architects of Fear: Conspiracy Theories and Paranoia in American Politics*. Los Angeles: Jeremy P. Tarcher: 1983.

Jones, Elwyn, ed. *Ripper File*. London: Barker, 1975.

Kahane, Claire. "Gothic Mirrors and Feminine Identity." *The Centennial Review* 24 (1980): 43–64.

Kaplan, Alice Yaeger. *Reproductions of Banality: Fascism, Literature, and French Intellectual Life*. Minneapolis: University of Minnesota Press, 1986.

Katz, Jacob. *From Prejudice to Destruction: Anti-Semitism, 1700–1933*. Cambridge, Mass.: Harvard University Press, 1980.

———. *Jews and Freemasons in Europe, 1723–1929*. Translated by Leonard Oschry. Cambridge, Mass.: Harvard University Press, 1970.

Kelly, Alexander. *Jack the Ripper: A Bibliography and Review of the Literature*. London: AAL, 1973.

Kennedy, Paul and Anthony Nicholls, eds. *Nationalist and Racialist Movements in Britain and Germany Before 1914*. Oxford: St. Anthony's / Macmillan, 1981.

Knight, Stephen. *Jack the Ripper: The Final Solution*. Chicago: Academy Chicago Publishers, 1986.

Krafft-Ebing, Richard von. *Psychopathia Sexualis: A Medico-Forensic Study*. 1886. Introduction by Dr. Ernest van den Haag. Reprint, New York: G. P. Putnam's, 1965.

Kristeva, Julia. *Powers of Horror: An Essay on Abjection*. Translated by Leon S. Roudiez. New York: Columbia University Press, 1982.

Lacoue-Labarthe, Philippe and Jean-Luc Nancy. "The Nazi Myth." *Critical Inquiry* 16 (winter 1990): 291–312.

Leatherdale, Clive. *Dracula: The Novel and the Legend*. Wellingborough, Northhamptonshire: Aquarian, 1985.

Levine, George and U. C. Knoepflmacher, eds. *The Endurance of Frankenstein: Essays on Mary Shelley's Novel*. Berkeley and Los Angeles: California University Press, 1979.

Livingston, Ira. "The Traffic in Leeches: David Cronenberg's *Rabid* and the Semiotics of Parasitism." *American Image* 50, no. 4 (winter 1993): 515–33.

Lombroso, Cesare. Introduction to *Criminal Man According to the Classifications of Cesare Lombroso*, by Gina Lombroso Ferrero. New York and London: 1911.

Marcus, Steven. *The Other Victorians: A Study of Sexuality and Pornography in Mid-Nineteenth-Century England*. New York: Basic, 1966.

Masse, Michelle A. *In the Name of Love: Women, Masochism and the Gothic*. Ithaca and London: Cornell University Press, 1992.

McCarty, John. *Splatter Movies: Breaking the Last Taboo of the Screen*. New York: St. Martin's, 1984.

McCormick, Donald. *The Identity of Jack the Ripper*. London: Arrow, 1970.

Mellor, Anne K. *Mary Shelley: Her Life, Her Fiction, Her Monsters*. New York and London: Routledge, 1988.

Miller, David A. *The Novel and the Police*. Berkeley and Los Angeles: University of California Press, 1988.

Moers, Ellen. *Literary Women*. London: The Women's Press, 1978.

Moretti, Franco. *Signs Taken for Wonders: Essays in the Sociology of Literary Form*. Translated by Susan Fischer, David Forgacs, and David Miller. London: Verso, 1983.

Mosse, George L. *Nationalism and Sexuality: Respectability and Abnormal Sexuality in Modern Europe*. New York: Howard Fertig, 1985.

———. *Toward the Final Solution: A History of European Racism*. New York: Howard Fertig, 1978.

Nicholson, Linda J., ed. *Feminism/Postmodernism*. New York and London: Routledge, 1990.

Nordau, Max Simon. *Degeneration*. London: D. Appleton and Co., 1895.

Punter, David. *The Literature of Terror: A History of Gothic Fictions from 1765 to the Present Day*. London and New York: Longman, 1980.

Ragussis, Michael. "The Birth of a Nation in Victorian Culture: The Spanish Inquisition, the Converted Daughter, and the 'Secret Race.'" *Critical Inquiry* 20 (spring 1994): 477–508.

Restuccia, Francis L. "Female Gothic Writing: 'Under Cover to Alice.'" *Genre* 19, no. 3 (fall 1986).

Rosenberg, Edgar. *From Shylock to Svengali: Jewish Stereotypes in English Fiction*. Stanford, Calif.: Stanford University Press, 1960.

Roth, Phyllis. "Suddenly Sexual Women in Bram Stoker's *Dracula*." *Literature and Psychology* 17, no. 3 (1977): 113–21.

Rumbelow, Donald. *The Complete Jack the Ripper*. New York: New American Library, 1975.

Sage, Victor. *Horror Fiction in the Protestant Tradition*. New York: St. Martin's, 1988.

Said, Edward. *Orientalism*. New York: Vintage, 1979.

Samuel, Maurice. *Blood Accusation: The Strange History of the Beiliss Case*. New York: Knopf, 1966.

Sedgwick, Eve Kosofsky. *Between Men: English Literature and Male Homosocial Desire*. New York: Columbia University Press, 1985.

——. *The Coherence of Gothic Conventions*. New York and London: Methuen, 1986.

——. *The Epistemology of the Closet*. Berkeley and Los Angeles: University of California Press, 1990.

Seitzer, Mark. "Serial Killing (1)." *differences: A Journal of Feminist Cultural Studies* 5, no. 1 (1993): 92–128.

Senf, Carole A. "*Dracula:* Stoker's Response to the New Woman." *Victorian Studies* 26 (1982).

Showalter, Elaine. *Sexual Anarchy: Gender and Culture at the Fin De Siècle*. New York: Viking, 1990.

——. "Syphilis, Sexuality, and the Fiction of the Fin de Siècle." In *Sex, Politics, and Science in the Nineteenth-Century Novel: Selected Papers from the English Institute 1983–4*, edited by Ruth Bernard Yeazell, 88–115. Baltimore and London: Johns Hopkins University Press, 1986.

Silverman, Kaja. *The Acoustic Mirror: The Female Voice in Psychoanalysis and Cinema*. Bloomington: Indiana University Press, 1988.

Sontag, Susan. *Illness as Metaphor*. New York: Vintage, 1978.

Stevenson, John Allen. "A Vampire in the Mirror: The Sexuality of *Dracula*." *PMLA* 103, no. 2 (March 1988): 139–49.

Stokes, John, ed. *Fin de Siècle/Fin du Globe: Fears and Fantasies of the Late Nineteenth Century*. New York: St. Martin's, 1992.

Stubbs, Patricia. *Women and Fiction: Feminism and the Novel, 1880–1920*. Sussex: Harvester, 1979.

Summers, Montague. *The Gothic Quest: A History of Gothic*. New York: Russell and Russell, 1938.

Tatar, Maria M. *Spellbound: Studies on Mesmerism and Literature*. Princeton, N.J.: Princeton University Press, 1978.

Theweleit, Klaus. *Male Fantasies*. Vol. 1, *Women, Floods, Bodies, History*. Translated by Stephen Conway with Erica Carter and Chris Turner. Minneapolis: University of Minnesota Press, 1987.

——. *Male Fantasies*. Vol. 2, *Male Bodies: Psychoanalyzing the White Terror*. Translated by Erica Carter and Chris Turner with Stephen Conway. Minneapolis: University of Minnesota Press, 1989.

Todorov, Tzvetan. *The Fantastic: A Structural Approach to the Genre*. Translated by Richard Howard. Ithaca, N.Y.: Cornell University Press, 1975.

Varma, Devendra P. "The Genesis of *Dracula:* A Re-Visit." *In Dracula: The Vampire and the Critics,* edited by Margaret Carter, 39–50. Ann Arbor and London: U.M.I. Research Press, 1988.

Varnado, S. L. *Haunted Presence: The Numinous in Gothic Fiction*. Tuscaloosa and London: The University of Alabama Press, 1987.

Vincinus, Martha. *Suffer and Be Still*. Bloomington: Indiana University Press, 1972.

Von Eckardt, Wolf, Sander L. Gilman, and J. Edward Chamberlain. *Oscar Wilde's London: A Scrapbook of Vices and Virtues, 1880–1900*. Garden City, N.J.: Doubleday and Co., 1987.

Walkowitz, Judith. "Jack the Ripper and the Myth of Male Violence." *Feminist Studies* 8, no. 3 (fall 1982).

——. *Prostitution and Victorian Society: Women, Class and the State*. New York: Cambridge University Press, 1980.

——. "Science, Feminism and Romance: The Men and Women's Club, 1885–1889." *History Workshop* 21 (spring 1986).

Waller, Gregory A., ed. *American Horrors: Essays on the Modern American Horror Film*. Urbana and Chicago: University of Illinois Press, 1987.

Weininger, Otto. *Sex and Character*. London: William Heinemann, 1906.

Weissman, Judith. "Bram Stoker: Semidemons and Secretaries." In *Half Savage and Hardy and Free*. Middletown, Conn.: Wesleyan University Press, 1987.

——. "Women and Vampires: *Dracula* as a Victorian Novel." *Midwest Quarterly* 18, no. 4 (summer 1977).

Williams, Linda. *Hard Core: Power, Pleasure and the "Frenzy of the Visible"*. Berkeley and Los Angeles: University of California Press, 1989.

——. "When the Woman Looks." in *Re-Visions: Essays in Feminist Film Criticism,* edited by Linda Williams, Mary Ann Doane, and Patricia Mellencamp. Frederick, Md.: University Publications of America, 1984.

Wilt, Judith. *Ghosts of the Gothic: Austen, Eliot, & Lawrence*. Princeton, N.J.: Princeton University Press, 1980.

Wolf, Leonard. *The Annotated Dracula*. New York: Clarkson N. Potter, 1975.

——. *The Annotated Frankenstein*. New York: Clarkson N. Potter, 1977.

Wolstenholme, Susan. *Gothic (Re)Visions: Writing Women as Readers*. Albany: State University of New York Press, 1993.

Young, Elizabeth. "*The Silence of the Lambs* and the Flaying of Feminist Theory." *Camera Obscura* 27 (September 1991): 4–35.

Žižek, Slavoj. "Grimaces of the Real, or When the Phallus Appears." *October* 58 (fall 1991): 44–68.

——. *The Sublime Object of Ideology*. London and New York: Verso, 1989.

Index

ABOUT THE AUTHOR
Judith Halberstam is Assistant Professor of Literature
at the University of California at San Diego.

Library of Congress Cataloging-in-Publication Data
Halberstam, Judith
Skin shows : gothic horror and the technology of monsters / Judith
Halberstam.
Includes bibliographical references and index.
ISBN 0-8223-1651-X (cl). — ISBN 0-8223-1663-3 (pa)
1. Horror tales, English — History and criticism. 2. Gothic
revival (Literature) — Great Britain. 3. Literature and technology —
Great Britain. 4. Horror films — History and criticism.
5. Monsters in motion pictures. 6. Monsters in literature.
I. Title.
PR830.T3H27   1995
823'.0872909 — dc20   95-948 CIP